your
pregnancy™
Quick Guide

Labor and Delivery

D1466578

your pregnancy™
Quick Guide

Labor and Delivery

What You Need to Know about Childbirth

Glade B. Curtis, M.D., M.P.H., OB-GYN
and Judith Schuler, M.S.

Da Capo
LIFE
LONG

A Member of the Perseus Books Group

Copyright 2004 © by Glade B. Curtis and Judith Schuler

Designed by Brent Wilcox
Set in 11.5-point Minion by The Perseus Books Group

Cataloging-in-Publication data for this book is available from the Library of Congress.

First printing, 2004
ISBN 0-7382-0969-4

Published by Da Capo Press
A Member of the Perseus Books Group
http://www.dacapopress.com

Note: The information in this book is true and complete to the best of our knowledge. The book is intended only as an informative guide for those wishing to know more about labor and delivery. In no way is this book intended to replace, countermand or conflict with the advice given to you by your physician. The ultimate decision concerning your care should be made between you and your doctors. We strongly recommend that you follow his or her advice. The information in this book is general and is offered with no guarantees on the part of the authors or Da Capo Press. The authors and publisher disclaim all liability in connection with the use of this book. The names and identifying details of people associated with events described in this book have been changed. Any similarity to actual persons is coincidental.

Da Capo Press books are available at special discounts for bulk purchases in the U.S. by corporations, institutions, and other organizations. For more information, please contact the Special Markets Department at the Perseus Books Group, 11 Cambridge Center, Cambridge, MA 02142, or call (800) 255-1514 or (617) 252-5298, or email special.markets@perseusbooks.com.

1 2 3 4 5 6 7 8 9—08 07 06 05 04

Find It Fast!

One of the greatest concerns pregnant women have is labor and delivery. It is unique, unlike any experience you have ever had before. You may be a little nervous about what's going to happen. That's natural. But be positive—this is a wonderful miracle for you and your partner.

You probably have lots of questions and concerns. Work with your doctor to make your labor and delivery a good experience. Learn what you need to know and to do to be prepared—ask about what will happen, the medications you might be offered, what prompts your doctor to do a C-section. Ask your doctor to tell you what you can do to have a healthy pregnancy. Discuss any concerns you may have. Below are some things you may want to consider as you progress through your pregnancy.

- Become informed about pregnancy and the birth experience. Knowledge is power. When you understand what can and will occur during labor and delivery, you may be able to relax more. Read our other pregnancy books, discuss questions and concerns with your doctor and share information and your knowledge with your partner.
- The relationships you have with your doctor and other members of your healthcare team are very important. Be an active member of the team by

following medical suggestions. Expect your medical team to work hard for you. Each of you should support the other.

- Being able to help make decisions about labor and delivery, including birth positions, pain-relief methods and your partner's level of participation in labor and delivery, helps you feel more in control. Discuss questions and various situations with your doctor at prenatal appointments.

The best advice we can give you before your labor begins is to relax. No one knows what's going to happen. Even medical professionals can be surprised by what occurs. Women have been having babies for a very long time, so you're not the first! Before you know it, you'll be holding the baby you've been waiting so long to meet. You may even say, "That wasn't so bad!"

Note: Throughout the book, you will find boxes titled "What Can I Do? How Can I Help?" for your partner. This is a time many expectant dads fear. They want to help but don't know how. Few know how they will handle the experience of labor and childbirth. Many men worry about their partner and how this whole situation will change their couple relationship. We offer tips, suggestions and ideas to help involve your partner more in this wondrous time you will share.

Part I: Getting Ready before Labor Begins

Preparing for Baby's Birth

- You may be feeling a little nervous about the birth. You might be afraid you won't know when it's time to call the doctor or go to the hospital.
- Don't hesitate to talk to your doctor about it at one of your visits. He or she will tell you what signs to watch for.
- In prenatal classes, you should also learn to recognize the signs of labor and when you should call your doctor or go to the hospital.
- Your bag of waters may break before you go into labor. In most cases, you'll notice this as a gush of water followed by a steady leaking. (See page 66.)
- During the last few weeks of pregnancy, have your suitcase packed and ready to go. See the discussion beginning on page 28 for some helpful suggestions. You'll have things you want at the hospital.
- Have insurance papers filled out and available.
- If you can, tour the hospital facilities a few weeks before your due date. Find out where to go and what happens when you get there.

- Talk with your partner about the best ways to reach him if you think you are in labor.
- Ask your doctor what you should do if you think you're in labor. Is it best to call the office? Should you go directly to the hospital? Should you call the answering service? By knowing what to do and when to do it, you'll be able to relax a little and not worry about the beginning of labor and delivery.
- It may be helpful and save time if you register at the hospital a few weeks before your due date. You can get forms at your doctor's office or from the hospital. It helps to do this before you go to the hospital in labor because you may be in a hurry and concerned with other things.
- You should know certain facts, including the following:
  - ~ your blood type and Rh-factor
  - ~ when your last period was and what your due date is
  - ~ details of any past pregnancies, including complications
  - ~ your doctor's name
  - ~ your pediatrician's name
- Signs that your labor may be about to begin include:
  - ~ increase of Braxton-Hicks contractions (see page 4)
  - ~ feeling the baby "drop" lower into your pelvis (see page 68)

~ weight loss or a break in weight gain
~ increased pressure in the pelvis and rectum
~ changes in vaginal discharge
~ diarrhea

Tips for the Expectant Dad *What Can I Do? How Can I Help?*

In the weeks before baby's birth, help your partner fill out all the forms she will be given—hospital forms, insurance forms and any other forms she receives. It's easier to fill them out together so you can each provide necessary personal data.

Keep Your Options Open during Labor and Delivery

When planning for your labor and delivery, think about the method(s) you may use to get through the process.

- Will you have epidural anesthesia?
- Are you going to attempt a drug-free delivery?
- Will you need an episiotomy?
- Every woman is different, and every labor is different. It's difficult to anticipate what will happen and what you will need during labor and delivery for pain relief.
- It's impossible to know how long labor will last— 3 hours or 20 hours.
- Make a flexible plan.

- Understand what's available and what options you can choose during labor.
- During the last 2 months of your pregnancy, discuss these concerns with your doctor and become familiar with his or her philosophy about labor.
- Know what can be provided for you at the hospital you've chosen. For example, some medications may not be available in your area or a pain-relief method may not be used at the hospital you choose.

Tips for the Expectant Dad

What Can I Do? How Can I Help?

Ask your partner to involve you in her plans for labor and delivery. Go to prenatal visits with her so the two of you can each ask the doctor questions about what will happen before, during and after labor and delivery.

Braxton-Hicks Contractions and False Labor

- *Braxton-Hicks contractions* are painless, nonrhythmical contractions you may be able to feel when you place your hand on your abdomen. These contractions often begin early in pregnancy and are felt at irregular intervals. They may increase in number and strength when the uterus is massaged. They are not positive signs of true labor.

- *False labor* often occurs before true labor begins. False-labor contractions can be painful and may feel like real labor to you. In most instances, false-labor contractions are irregular. They are usually of short duration (less than 45 seconds). Discomfort may occur in various parts of your body, such as the groin, lower abdomen or back.
- False labor is usually seen in late pregnancy. It seems to occur more often in women who have been pregnant before and delivered more babies. It usually stops as quickly as it begins. There doesn't appear to be any danger to you or your baby.
- With *true labor*, uterine contractions produce pain that starts at the top of the uterus and radiates over the entire uterus, through the lower back into the pelvis. Ask your doctor what the signs of labor contractions are; they are usually regular.
- Contractions increase in duration and strength over time. You'll notice a regular rhythm to real labor contractions.
- You'll want to time contractions so you know how frequently they occur and how long they last. When you go to the hospital depends in part on your contractions.

True Labor or False Labor?

Considerations	True Labor	False Labor
Contractions	Regular	Irregular
Time between contractions	Come closer together	Do not get closer together
Contraction intensity	Increases	Doesn't change
Location of contractions	Entire abdomen	Various locations or back
Effect of anesthetic or pain relievers	Will not stop labor	Sedation may stop or alter frequency of pain
Cervical change	Progressive cervical change	No cervical change

Childbirth-Education Classes

You and your partner can be better prepared for what lies ahead if you take a birth-preparation course. About 90% of all first-time expectant parents take some type of class. Women who take childbirth classes need less medication, have fewer forceps deliveries and feel more positive about birth than women who don't take classes.

- The goal of a class is to provide you with information so you can be prepared to make the best, most well-informed decisions during your labor and delivery.
- If you're better prepared, you'll be more at ease during labor and delivery.

- The list below can help you evaluate whether a childbirth-education class is right for you as a couple.
  - ~ Class was recommended by your doctor or his or her office staff.
  - ~ Class uses a philosophy shared by your doctor.
  - ~ Class begins when you need it, around the 7th month of pregnancy.
  - ~ Class size is small—no more than 10 or 12 couples—and classroom is large enough to allow you the opportunity to practice (on the floor) what you learn in class.
  - ~ Class includes a tour of the hospital and the labor and delivery areas (if it is a hospital-sponsored class).
  - ~ Graduates are enthusiastic. (Locate some, and ask about the class.)
  - ~ Class is candid about the birth experience. Pain during labor and delivery is *not* glossed over or downplayed.
  - ~ Class covers inducing labor, Cesarean delivery, episiotomies and different types of pain-relief methods.
  - ~ You get to view videos of an actual birth and a C-section.
  - ~ Information is provided about postpartum distress, circumcision and feeding baby.

~ Class includes the time and the opportunity to ask questions, practice techniques and talk to parents who have recently given birth.

~ Class involves doctors (anesthesiologists, pediatricians) and/or nurses.

- Most childbirth-education classes run 4 to 6 weeks— you and your labor coach attend one class each week.

- If you can't find the time in your schedules to attend this many classes, consider an all-day class or a weekend class. A short class is better than no class!

- Or consider private, individualized sessions in your home. An instructor comes to you, when you are free; classes can be as long or as short as your schedules permit.

- Sign up for your class early in the second trimester, so you'll be sure to have a place, and you'll be able to finish it before your due date.

- Practice what you learn in your classes.

- If you can't find a way to go to classes, at least take a tour of the hospital or birthing center you have chosen. It'll help you feel more comfortable when it's time for baby to be born.

- Check out the qualifications of the person teaching the class (most are women). Also see page 14.

- Some instructors are medically trained, such as a labor-and-delivery nurse; others have no medical training at all.

- Once you have found a class you think will work for you, find out how long it lasts, how much it costs, what the class curriculum includes, the instructor's credentials and the childbirth philosophy of the class (is there just one?).
- Then you and your partner will be able to decide whether a particular class is just right for you!

What Will You Learn in a Class?

- By meeting in class on a regular basis, you can learn about many things that concern you.
- Classes are intended to help you and your partner or labor coach learn about pregnancy, what happens at the hospital and what happens during labor and delivery.
- Some couples find classes are a good way to get a partner more involved and to help make him feel more comfortable with the pregnancy, labor and delivery.
- Classes may give your partner the opportunity to take a more active part during your pregnancy and at the time of labor and delivery.
- Classes often cover a wide range of subjects, including the following areas.
  - ~ What are the different childbirth methods?
  - ~ What is "natural childbirth"?

~ What is a Cesarean delivery?

~ What pain-relief methods are available?

~ What you need to know (and to practice) for the childbirth method you choose.

~ Is an episiotomy always necessary?

~ What are the benefits of an enema?

~ When is a fetal monitor necessary?

~ What happens when you reach the hospital?

~ Is an epidural or some other type of anesthesia right for you?

~ In addition, your class may provide you information about lactation consultants, doulas, other types of care and additional resources you may find valuable.

• A class is also a great way to connect with other expectant couples.

Tips for the Expectant Dad
What Can I Do? How Can I Help?

Childbirth-education classes are good for you both—if your partner asks you to attend the classes, go! Together you will learn many things that can help you during labor and delivery. Information is also provided about the days and weeks after baby's birth, so you can get a good start at being a dad.

Who Goes to Prenatal Classes?

- Classes are usually held for small groups of pregnant women and their partners or labor coaches. It helps to be able to interact with other couples and to ask questions. It's also comforting to know other couples are concerned about many of the same things you are, such as labor and pain management. It's good to know you aren't the only one thinking about what lies ahead.
- Prenatal classes are not only for couples who are pregnant for the first time. If you have a new partner, if it has been a few years since you've had a baby, if you have questions or if you would like a review of what lies ahead, a prenatal class can help you.
- These classes may help reduce worry or concern you and your partner feel about labor and delivery. They'll help you enjoy the birth of your baby even more.

Where Do You Take the Classes?

- Childbirth classes are offered in many places.
- Most hospitals that deliver babies offer prenatal classes, often taught by labor-and-delivery nurses or by a midwife.

- If you take a class taught by the hospital personnel where you will give birth, you'll learn about the hospital's policies and services.
- Hospital classes often offer tours of the maternity ward and the nursery.
- These classes are often quite large, so you may not get a lot of personal attention.
- In addition, hospital classes may not fully discuss non-drug pain management and relaxation techniques.
- Independent classes—those that are not affiliated with a hospital—are taught in a variety of settings, from churches to community centers.
- These classes may be smaller in size, so you will receive a lot more individual attention. They often cover a wide range of topics.
- Some classes have different degrees of involvement.
- The time commitment and/or depth of a subject covered is different for each of the various classes that may be available.
- Ask at the doctor's office about classes they recommend. They can help you decide which type of class would be best for you.

Different Childbirth Programs

Some women decide before the birth of their baby that they are going to labor and deliver with *natural childbirth*. The description or definition of natural childbirth varies from one couple to another.

- Many people equate natural childbirth with a drug-free labor and delivery.
- Others equate natural childbirth with the use of mild pain medications or local pain medications, such as numbing medications in the area of the vagina for delivery or for an episiotomy and repair of episiotomy.
- Most agree that natural childbirth is birth with as few artificial procedures as possible.
- A woman who chooses natural childbirth usually needs some advance instruction to prepare for it.
- Childbirth preparation methods are usually divided among three major programs—Lamaze, Bradley and Grantly Dick-Read. Each program offers its own techniques and methods.
  - ~ *Lamaze* is the oldest technique of childbirth preparation; about 25% of all pregnant women in America take these courses. Lamaze emphasizes relaxation and breathing as ways to ease pain during labor and delivery. Partners are included in Lamaze classes.
  - ~ *Bradley* classes teach relaxation and inward focus; many types of relaxation are used. Bradley classes often begin when pregnancy is confirmed and continue until after the birth. Women in Bradley classes usually do not want to use any type of medication for labor-pain relief.

~ *Grantly Dick-Read* is a method that attempts to break the fear-tension-pain cycle of labor and delivery through training and practice of particular techniques. These classes were the first to include fathers in the birth experience.

- Other groups also offer classes.

~ The *Association of Labor Assistants and Childbirth Educators (ALACE)* holds classes that teach relaxation methods to help a woman through the pain and discomfort of giving birth.

~ *Birth Works, Inc.,* is an organization whose goal is to help women undergo more-positive birth experiences by learning to trust more in their own instincts about their bodies.

~ *The International Childbirth Education Association (ICEA)* doesn't advocate any particular birth program or take a stand regarding pain relief during birth. They provide information to help a couple make choices based on their knowledge of alternatives.

The Childbirth-Education Class Instructor

- A class—no matter where it is taught—is only as good as its instructor.
- Unfortunately, there is no licensing for instructors, although a number of organizations do certify people to act as instructors.

- Check out the instructor's credentials *before* you sign up for a class.
- Some "certified" instructors earned credentials by attending a seminar that lasted for several days to a week.
- Other instructors have completed a 2-year program, including an apprenticeship.

Choosing Your Class

- Begin looking into classes that are offered in your area around 20 weeks of pregnancy.
- Ask your doctor or the office nurse to recommend classes in your area.
- Friends can also be good sources.
- Or look in the yellow pages under "Childbirth Education."
- You may have to sign up early. Classes should start by the beginning of the 3rd trimester (about 27 weeks).
- Try to finish the classes at least a few weeks before your due date.
- The cost of classes can range from $50 to over $300 (for private instruction).
- In some areas, classes are free.
- Some insurance companies and some HMOs pay part or all of the class fees.
- It's important to practice what you learn in your classes.

- Try to practice for at least 20 minutes a day or as much as the instructor suggests.
- If you can't practice 20 minutes a day, four 30-minute sessions each week should be beneficial.
- If you don't practice what you learn, it will be harder to put into action during labor and delivery the things you learn in class.

Tips for the Expectant Dad *What Can I Do? How Can I Help?*

Encourage your partner to practice what you learn in your classes. Set aside some time every night so the two of you can review all the new material. If you practice together now, you'll have it all down pat when you really need it!

Can You Take Prenatal Classes If You Have Problems?

- If you have problems getting to a prenatal class because of cost or time or because you're on bed rest, it may be possible to take classes at home.
- You might also consider *Great Expectations: Laugh and Learn About Childbirth*. This is a two-videotape set that may provide you with a lot of the information you would learn in a class. The set is available

for $65, including shipping and handling; call 877-715-2844 or visit www.laughandlearn.com for further information.

Who Will Be Your Labor Coach?

- You probably want your partner to be your labor coach. Although it is nice for your partner to act as your coach, it's not mandatory.
- It's not unusual for a man to have some fear or dread about participating in the birth.
- Ask your partner if he wants to be your coach. If he doesn't, try to accept it. Some men are not able to cope with labor and delivery.
- Ask him what he *is* willing to do—from sitting in the waiting room to participating in a limited way, such as standing next to you and holding your hand.
- You can choose a friend or family member to act as your coach.

What Does the Labor Coach Do?

A good labor coach can help make the birth experience positive and rewarding. It helps your labor coach if you tell him or her what you need and want. You'll both need to be flexible. During labor, a situation can quickly change, and a new plan may need to be put into motion. A labor coach is your advocate. He or she should inform the hospital staff when you are in pain or when labor activity changes, keep out unwanted visitors and ask for items you need. Your labor coach also:

- helps time contractions
- assists you in your breathing techniques
- knows which technique is appropriate for different stages of labor
- listens to the labor nurse who may offer excellent advice, based on experience
- offers you ice chips or a damp washcloth if you become dehydrated
- tries to distract you when the time seems right
- helps make you more comfortable
- offers to massage your sore back or aching muscles
- lets you make major decisions about aspects of the birth, such as whether you need pain medication
- guards your privacy
- doesn't take things personally; ignores it if you get touchy or seem angry
- doesn't leave the labor room to make phone calls for work; doesn't take work into the labor room
- doesn't leave without letting someone know where he or she is going

- gives you the attention you want; leaves you alone when you don't want it
- doesn't take pictures if you ask him or her not to

Tips for the Expectant Dad

What Can I Do? How Can I Help?

Be honest with your partner if you *really* do not want to be her labor coach or if there are issues related to labor and delivery that scare you. She may be disappointed, but it's better for you to be open with her about your discomfort. That way she can find someone else to act as her coach, and you can avoid an embarrassing situation in the delivery room. You can still be involved in the birth experience, even if it's just stroking her hair or holding her hand to let her know you are there for her.

Even if your partner decides he can't be your labor coach, he can still be involved in the birth experience. He can:

- time your contractions so you are both aware of labor's progress
- encourage and reassure you during labor
- help create a mood in the labor room
- support you in any way you ask him to
- protect privacy for both of you, control who visits and when, and oversee telephone calls
- report to family members how labor is progressing

- play music, read or distract you in some other way
- cut the baby's umbilical cord after the birth

Being together can help you both during this wondrous time. Sharing in the joy of your baby's birth can begin your bonding experience as a family.

What Is a Doula?

- A *doula* is a woman who is trained to provide support and assistance to a pregnant woman during labor and delivery of her baby. She is a professional labor assistant.
- A doula is different from a midwife because a doula does not deliver babies.
- A doula remains with the woman from the onset of labor until her baby is born.
- Doulas provide physical and emotional support when a woman chooses to have a drug-free labor and delivery. She can also provide hands-on comfort during labor and delivery.
- Support from a doula can range from giving you a massage to helping you focus on your breathing.
- She may even be able to help you begin breastfeeding your baby.
- A doula assists the labor coach. She does not displace or replace a labor coach; she works with him or her.

- Your partner can still play a vital role; a doula can take some of the pressure off his shoulders.
- In some situations, a doula may *serve* as the labor coach.
- The services of a doula may be expensive and can range from $250 to $1500. This covers labor and one or more prenatal visits. Insurance does not pay for this service.
- If you and your partner choose to have a doula present during labor and the birth, talk to your doctor about your decision. He or she may find her presence intrusive and veto the idea. Or the doctor may be able to give you the name of someone he or she often works with.
- If you decide you want a doula, begin looking for one early in your pregnancy.
- If you have decided you want anesthesia, no matter what, a doula may not be a wise choice for you.

Kick Count

Toward the end of pregnancy, you may be asked to record how often you feel your baby move. This test is done at home and is called a *kick count*. It provides reassurance about fetal well-being; this information is similar to that learned by a nonstress test. (See the discussion of the nonstress test on page 31.) Your doctor may use one of two common methods.

- The first method is to count how many times the baby moves in an hour.
- The second method is to note how long it takes baby to move 10 times.
- Usually you can choose when you want to do the test.
- After eating a meal is a good time to count kicks because baby is often more active then.

Choosing Where to Give Birth

- There may be many options for you, when it comes to choosing where to give birth.
- In some situations, you may not have a choice. Or you may have several choices in your area.
- Whatever birthing setup you choose, the most important considerations are the health of your baby and the welfare of you both.
- When you decide where to have your baby, be sure you have answered the following questions, if you can.
  - ~ What facilities and staff do you have available?
  - ~ What is the availability of anesthesia? Is an anesthesiologist available 24 hours a day?

~ How long does it take them to respond and to perform a Cesarean delivery, if necessary? (This should be 30 minutes or less.)

~ Is a pediatrician available 24 hours a day for an emergency or problems?

~ Is the nursery staffed at all times?

~ In the event of an emergency or a premature baby that needs to be transported to a high-risk nursery, how is it done? By ambulance? By helicopter?

~ How close is the nearest high-risk nursery, if not at this hospital?

~ Does my insurance cover this choice?

• These may seem like a lot of questions to ask, but the answers can help put your mind at ease.

• When it's your baby and your health, it's good to know emergency measures can be employed in an efficient, timely manner when necessary.

Tips for the Expectant Dad
What Can I Do? How Can I Help?

Wherever you and your partner choose for your baby's birth, know how to get there and find out where to go at the hospital. Plan a few alternate routes, if there is more than one way to get to where you're going. Drive each one at least once, adding time for bad weather if that could be a factor at the time of delivery.

LDRP (Labor, Delivery, Recovery and Postpartum)

- With LDRP (labor, delivery, recovery and post-partum), the room you are admitted to at the beginning of your labor is the room you labor in, deliver in, recover in and remain in for your entire hospital stay.
- The concept of LDRP has evolved because many women don't want to be moved from the labor area to delivery, then to recovery, then to another part of the hospital for the rest of their stay.
- The nursery is usually close to labor and delivery and the recovery area so you can see your baby as often as you like and have your baby in your room for longer periods.
- LDRP isn't available everywhere, but these facilities are becoming more popular.

Labor-and-Delivery Suite

- In some places, you will labor in a labor-and-delivery suite, then be moved to a delivery room at the time of delivery.

- Following this, you may go to a postpartum floor, which is an area in the hospital where you will spend the remainder of your stay.
- Most hospitals allow you to have your baby in your room as much as you want.
- This is called *rooming in* or *boarding in.* Some hospitals also have a cot, couch or chair that makes into a bed in your room so your partner can stay with you after delivery.
- If you're interested, check the availability of various facilities in the hospitals in your area. And check to see if they are covered by your insurance.

Birthing Room

- Another option is the birthing room; this generally refers to delivering your baby in the same room you labor in. In some areas, it is called *LDR (labor, delivery and recovery).*
- You don't have to be moved from the room you're laboring in to another place to have the baby.
- Even if you use a birthing room, you may have to move to another area of the hospital for recovery and the remainder of your stay, which can be an advantage. You go to a clean room, where it may be quieter and more restful.

Is Home Birth Safe?

- You may have heard from friends or acquaintances that they had a home birth and everything went fine.
- In the recent past, there has been a growing interest in giving birth at home; some women feel giving birth at home is "more natural."
- Another factor in this decision may be the high cost of labor and delivery, especially if you don't have full insurance coverage.
- We do *not* recommend giving birth at home; it is an extremely risky undertaking.
- One study showed twice as many infant deaths and serious, dangerous complications when babies are delivered at home.
- There were also dangers to the mom—first-time pregnant women who delivered at home had nearly triple the risk of complications following the birth.
- The chance of serious problems increased when the woman suffered from gestational diabetes or high blood pressure or when she carried more than one baby.
- The American College of Obstetricians and Gynecologists (ACOG) has firmly stated that home birthing is hazardous to a woman and her baby.
- If you are interested in a more natural setting for your baby's birth, discuss it with your doctor. He or

she may be able to give you some suggestions to make your baby's birth at the hospital a more natural experience for you.

How Much Does Your Baby Weigh?

- You have probably asked your doctor several times how big your baby is or how much your baby will weigh when it's born. Next to asking about the sex of a baby, this is the most frequently asked question.
- Ultrasound can be used to estimate fetal weight. The accuracy of predicting fetal weight using ultrasound has improved.
- Several measurements are used in a formula or put in a computer program to estimate a baby's weight.
- Many feel that ultrasound is the method of choice to estimate fetal weight. But even with ultrasound, estimates may vary as much as half a pound or more in either direction.

Will Your Baby Fit through the Birth Canal?

- Even with a fetal-weight estimate, whether by your doctor or by ultrasound, we can't tell if the baby is too big for you or whether you'll need a C-section.

- Usually it's necessary for labor to begin before we are able to see how the baby fits into your pelvis and if there is room for it to pass through the birth canal.
- In some women who appear to be average or better-than-average size, a 6- or 6½-pound baby won't fit through the pelvis.
- Experience has also shown that women who may appear petite are sometimes able to deliver 7½-pound or larger babies without much difficulty.
- The best test or method of evaluating whether your baby will deliver through your pelvis is labor.

Packing for the Hospital

Packing for the hospital is important. Don't pack too early, but don't wait till the last minute. It's probably a good idea to pack about 3 weeks before your due date. This allows you time to think about what you want to take with you. Packing early also allows you to be ready if you go into labor early. This helps you avoid "panic packing," including items you don't need while forgetting more important ones.

- Pack things you'll need and your labor coach will need.
- Also pack things you and the baby will need after delivery, as well as for the hospital stay.

- Consider the following things for packing in your hospital bag:
  - ~ completed insurance or preregistration forms and insurance card
  - ~ heavy socks to wear in the delivery room
  - ~ an item to use as a focal point
  - ~ 1 cotton nightgown or T-shirt for labor
  - ~ lip balm, lollipops or fruit drops, to use during labor
  - ~ light diversion, such as books or magazines, to use during labor
  - ~ breath spray
  - ~ 1 or 2 nightgowns for after labor (bring a nursing gown if you're going to breastfeed)
  - ~ slippers with rubber soles
  - ~ 1 long robe for walking in the halls
  - ~ 2 bras (nursing bras and pads if you breastfeed)
  - ~ 3 pairs of panties
  - ~ toiletries you use, including brush, comb, toothbrush, toothpaste, soap, shampoo, conditioner
  - ~ hairband or ponytail holder, if you have long hair
  - ~ loose-fitting clothes for going home
  - ~ sanitary pads, if the hospital doesn't supply them
  - ~ one or two pieces of fruit to eat after the delivery—don't pack them too early!
- You might want to include some things in your hospital kit for your partner or labor coach to help

you both during the birth. You might bring the following:

~ a watch with a second hand

~ talc or cornstarch for massaging you during labor

~ a paint roller or tennis ball for giving you a low-back massage during labor

~ tapes or CDs and a player, or a radio to play during labor

~ camera and film

~ list of telephone numbers and a long-distance calling card

~ change for telephones and vending machines

~ snacks for your partner or labor coach

- The hospital will probably supply most of what you need for your baby, but you might want to bring some of the following things:

~ clothes for the trip home, including an under-shirt, sleeper, outer clothes (a hat if it's cold outside)

~ a couple of baby blankets

~ diapers, if your hospital doesn't supply them

- You need an approved infant car seat in which to take your baby home. It's important to start your baby in a car seat the very first time he or she rides in a car! Many hospitals will not let you take your baby home without one.

Tips for the Expectant Dad

What Can I Do? How Can I Help?

It's a good idea for you to pack a hospital bag for yourself. Include a change of clothes, some reading materials (for when you can't be with your partner), a few snacks and anything else you might need to make yourself more comfortable.

Some Tests You May Have before the Birth

The Nonstress Test (NST)

- A nonstress test is a simple, noninvasive procedure done at 32 weeks of pregnancy or later.
- The test is performed in the doctor's office or in the labor-and-delivery department at the hospital.
- It measures how the fetal heart responds to the fetus's own movements and evaluates fetal well-being in late pregnancy.
- Doctors use the findings from the NST to help them evaluate how well a baby is tolerating life inside the uterus.
- The nonstress test is commonly used in overdue and high-risk pregnancies.
- While you are lying down, a technician attaches a fetal monitor (Doppler ultrasound) to your abdomen.

- Every time you feel your baby move, you push a button to make a mark on a strip of monitor paper. At the same time, the monitor records the baby's heartbeat.
- When the baby moves, its heart rate usually goes up.
- If the baby doesn't move or if the fetal heart rate does not react to movement, the test is called *nonreactive.*
- When baby doesn't move, it doesn't necessarily mean there is a problem—the baby may be sleeping.
- To help make baby move, you may be given something to eat or drink.
- If the baby still doesn't move, a buzzer that creates a sound and vibration to wake up the fetus may be used to make it move. This is called *vibration stimulation.*
- In more than 75% of nonreactive tests (not reassuring), the baby is healthy.
- However, a nonreactive test might be a sign the baby is not receiving enough oxygen or is experiencing some other problem.
- In this case, the test will probably be repeated in 24 hours, or additional tests will be ordered, including a contraction-stress test or a biophysical profile. See the discussions that follow.
- This test takes from 20 minutes to 45 minutes to complete.
- Your doctor will decide if further action is necessary.

Tips for the Expectant Dad
What Can I Do? How Can I Help?

If your partner must have any of these tests before baby's birth, try to go with her. She probably could use your moral support, and she'll appreciate your involvement. Occasionally a test will trigger labor; you wouldn't want to miss your baby's birth!

The Contraction-Stress Test (CST)

- If the nonstress test is nonreactive (see the discussion above), a contraction-stress test, also called a *stress test,* may be ordered.
- This test measures the response of the fetal heart to mild uterine contractions that mimic labor.
- It gives an indication of how the baby is doing and how well the baby might tolerate contractions and labor.
- If you have had a problem pregnancy in the past or if you experienced medical problems during this pregnancy, your doctor may order this test in the last few weeks of pregnancy.
- If you have diabetes and take insulin, your baby may be at some increased risk of problems. In that situation, the test may be done every week, beginning around 32 weeks.

- In some cases, the doctor may order the nonstress test alone or order both the nonstress test and the contraction-stress test at the same time. (The contraction-stress test is considered more accurate than the nonstress test.)
- A contraction-stress test is usually done in the hospital because it occasionally triggers labor.
- Three contractions must be recorded in about 10 minutes; each contraction must last about 40 seconds.
- The test can take as long as 2 hours to complete.
- A nurse places a monitor on your abdomen to record the fetal heart rate.
- You are attached to an I.V. that dispenses small amounts of the hormone oxytocin to make your uterus contract.
- Or nipple stimulation may be used to make your uterus contract.
- When the uterus contracts, the blood flow to the placenta decreases.
- If the baby is having trouble or the placenta isn't working well, the contraction can decrease the oxygen supply to the baby. This can cause the fetal heart rate to drop.
- The baby's heartbeat is monitored for its response to the contractions.

- The results of the test can be classified as *negative, positive, unsatisfactory* or *equivocal.*
- A negative test is good.
- A positive test is not good.
- Unsatisfactory or equivocal results mean the test was neither positive nor negative.
- Test results can indicate how well a baby might tolerate contractions and labor.
- If the baby doesn't respond well to contractions, it can be a sign of fetal stress.
- A slowed heart rate after a contraction is nonreassuring. This means the baby's status is not reassuring.
- The doctor may recommend delivery of the baby, if a CST is not reassuring.
- In other cases, the test may be repeated the next day, or a biophysical profile may be ordered. (See the discussion below.)
- If the test shows no sign of a slowed fetal heart rate, the test result is reassuring.
- Some believe this test is more accurate than the nonstress test in evaluating a baby's well-being.

Biophysical Profile

- A biophysical profile is an in-depth test to examine the baby during the last 2 months of pregnancy.

- It helps determine fetal health and is done when there is need for reassurance about the baby or there is concern about fetal well-being. The test evaluates the well-being of your baby inside your uterus.
- The test is usually done in high-risk situations, overdue pregnancies or pregnancies in which the baby doesn't move very much.
- It's also useful in evaluating an infant with intrauterine-growth restriction (IUGR).
- A biophysical profile uses a particular scoring system. The first four of the five tests listed below are made with ultrasound; the fifth is done with external fetal monitors.
- A biophysical profile is a nonstress test combined with ultrasound evaluations.
- A score is given to each of the five areas of evaluation, which include:
  ~ fetal breathing movements—even though the baby doesn't actually breathe air, the chest wall does move in and out
  ~ fetal body movements
  ~ fetal tone
  ~ amount of amniotic fluid (amniotic-fluid volume)
  ~ reactive fetal heart rate (nonstress test)
- Fetal "breathing" involves the movement or expansion of the baby's chest inside the uterus. This score is based on the amount of chest movement that occurs.

- Movement of the baby's body is noted. A normal score indicates normal body movements. An abnormal score is given when there are few or no body movements during the allotted time period.

- Fetal tone is evaluated similarly. Movement, or lack of movement, of baby's arms and legs is rated.

- Evaluation of the amount of amniotic fluid requires experience in ultrasound examination. A normal pregnancy has adequate fluid around the baby. An abnormal test indicates little or no amniotic fluid around the baby.

- Fetal heart-rate monitoring (nonstress test) is done with external monitors. It evaluates changes in the fetal heart rate associated with movement of the baby. The amount of change and number of changes in the fetal heart rate differ, depending on who is doing the test and their definition of normal.

- Evaluation may vary depending on the sophistication of the equipment used and the expertise of the person doing the test.

- For each test, a normal score is 2; an abnormal score is 0. A score of 1 in any of the tests is a middle score.

- From these five scores, a total score is obtained by adding all the values together.

- The higher the score, the better the baby's condition. A lower score may cause concern about the well-being of the fetus.

- A score of 8 to 10 is reassuring; 4 or less is not reassuring.
- If the score is low, a recommendation may be made to deliver the baby.
- If the score is reassuring, the test may be repeated at a later date.
- If results fall in the middle, the test may be repeated the following day, depending on the circumstances of the pregnancy.
- The test takes 30 to 40 minutes.
- Your doctor will evaluate all the information before making any decision.

Evaluating Baby's Lungs

- The respiratory system is the last fetal system to mature.
- Premature infants often have respiratory difficulties because their lungs are not fully developed.
- Knowing how mature a baby's lungs are helps the doctor make a decision about early delivery, if that must be considered.
- If the baby needs to be delivered early, tests can predict whether the baby will be able to breathe without assistance (lungs are mature).

- There are several fetal lung maturity tests available, including:
  - ~ lecithin/sphingomyelin ratio (L/S ratio)
  - ~ phosphatidyl glycerol (PG)
  - ~ foam stability index
  - ~ fluorescence polarization
  - ~ optical density at 650nm
  - ~ lamellar body counts
  - ~ saturated phosphatidylcholine
- The test a doctor chooses to use depends on availability and the experience of those taking care of the pregnant woman.
- Two tests used most often to evaluate a baby's lungs before birth are the *L/S ratio* and the *phosphatidyl glycerol (PG)* tests.
- Fluid for these two tests is obtained by amniocentesis.

Tips for the Expectant Dad *What Can I Do? How Can I Help?*

When you can, go to prenatal appointments with your partner. She may be having a hard time getting around on her own right now. Getting in and out of the car—even driving!—can be a hassle. She'll see you as her knight in shining armor if you're there to take care of her in the final weeks of her pregnancy.

Pelvic Exam in Late Pregnancy

- Toward the end of your pregnancy, around 36 weeks (or about 4 weeks before your due date), your doctor may do a pelvic exam. This pelvic exam helps your doctor evaluate the progress of your pregnancy. One of the first things he or she will observe is whether you are leaking amniotic fluid. If you think you are, it's important to tell your doctor.

- Your doctor will examine your cervix at the pelvic exam. During labor, the cervix usually becomes softer and thins out, called *effacement.*

- Your doctor will evaluate changes in your cervix for its softness or firmness and the amount of thinning.

- Before labor begins, your cervix is thick and is "0% effaced." It has not thinned out.

- When you're in active labor, the cervix thins out; when it is half-thinned, it is "50% effaced."

- Immediately before delivery, the cervix is "100% effaced" or completely thinned out.

- The dilatation (amount of opening) of the cervix is also important. This is usually measured in centimeters.

- The cervix is fully open when the diameter of the cervical opening measures 10cm. The goal is to be a 10!

- Before labor begins, the cervix may be closed. Or it may be open a little, such as 1cm (nearly ½ inch).

- The goal of labor is to stretch and open the cervix so the baby can fit through it and can pass out of the uterus.
- Your doctor also evaluates whether the baby's head, bottom or legs are coming first. (He or she may refer to a "presenting part.")
- The shape of your pelvic bones is also noted.
- The station is then determined. *Station* describes the degree to which the presenting part of the baby has descended into the birth canal.
- The 0 point is a bony landmark in the pelvis, the starting place of the birth canal. The birth canal is like a tube going from the pelvic girdle down through the pelvis and out the vagina. The baby travels through this tube from the uterus.
- If the baby's head is at a −2 station, it means the head is higher inside you than if it were at a +2 station.
- If you dilate during labor but the baby doesn't move down through the pelvis, a C-section may be needed because the baby's head doesn't fit through the pelvic girdle.

What Can Your Doctor Tell from a Pelvic Exam?

- When your doctor examines you by doing a pelvic exam, he or she may describe your situation in medical terms. You might hear something like "2cm, 50% and a –2 station," as described above.

- This means the cervix is open 2cm (about 1 inch), it is halfway thinned out (50% effaced) and the presenting part (baby's head, feet or buttocks) is at a –2 station.
- Try to remember this information, or write it down.
- You can tell the medical personnel in labor and delivery what your dilatation and effacement were at your last checkup so they can determine if your situation has changed if you go in for a labor check.

Premature Birth

- *Preterm birth* refers to a baby born before 37 weeks of gestation; it is also called *premature birth.*
- About 10% of all babies are born prematurely.
- Premature birth increases the risk of problems in the baby.
- Babies born prematurely usually weigh less than 5 pounds.
- In 1950, the neonatal death rate was about 20 per 1000 live births.

- Today, the rate is less than 10 per 1000 live births. Nearly twice the number of preterm infants survive today compared to 50 years ago.
- The decreasing death rate applies primarily to infants delivered during the 3rd trimester (27 weeks of pregnancy or more) who weigh at least 2¼ pounds and are without birth defects.
- When gestational age and birthweight are below these levels, the death rate increases.
- Better methods of caring for premature babies have contributed to higher survival statistics.
- Today, infants born as early as 25 weeks of pregnancy may survive.
- Recent information indicates the survival rate for infants who weighed between 1 pound and 1½ pounds is about 43%. For babies weighing between 1½ pounds and 2¼ pounds, the survival rate is about 72%.
- The average hospital stay for premature babies ranges from 125 days for infants weighing between 1⅓ and 1½ pounds to 76 days for babies in the 2- to 2¼-pound birthweight range.
- This discussion must include the frequency rate of problems these premature babies suffer.
- In the lower-birthweight range, many babies who survived had disabilities.

- Higher-weight babies also had disabilities, but statistics for this group were much lower.
- Preterm delivery of a baby can be serious because a baby's lungs and other systems may not be ready to function on their own.
- It's usually best for the baby to remain in the uterus as long as possible, so it can grow and develop fully.
- Your doctor may take steps to halt contractions if you go into labor too early.
- Follow all instructions from your doctor to help deal with this serious problem.
- Most doctors start with bed rest and increased fluids to stop labor.
- Bed rest means lying on your side in bed. Either side is OK, but the left side is best.
- Some medications may help stop labor.

Tips for the Expectant Dad
What Can I Do? How Can I Help?

If your partner experiences the symptoms of premature labor, help her follow her doctor's instructions. Support her if she has to stop working. If she's told bed rest is best, help her by doing chores around the house, cleaning up after yourself, making meals and doing the shopping and other household chores. If she has to go into the hospital to deal with the problem, tell her you'll take care of getting things ready for the baby. Give her encouragement, then follow through with your promises.

Causes of Premature
Labor and Premature Birth

- In most cases, the causes of premature labor and premature birth are unknown.
- Causes we do understand include a uterus with an abnormal shape, multiple fetuses, too much amniotic fluid, placental abruption, placenta previa, vasa previa, premature rupture of membranes, an incompetent cervix, abnormalities of the fetus, fetal death, a retained IUD, serious maternal illness or incorrect estimate of gestational age.
- Finding the cause of premature labor and delivery may be difficult.
- An attempt is always made to determine what causes preterm labor before active labor begins. In this way, treatment may be more effective.

Tests for Premature Labor

- One test, called *SalEst,* can help determine if a woman might go into labor too early.
- The test measures levels of the hormone estriol in a pregnant woman's saliva.
- There may be a surge in this chemical several weeks before early labor.

- A positive result means a woman has a 7 times higher chance of delivering her baby before the 37th week of pregnancy.
- Another test your doctor may do is a *fetal fibronectin (fFN) test.*
- Fetal fibronectin is a protein found in vaginal secretions up to about 20 weeks of pregnancy.
- If a doctor believes you may be going into premature labor, he or she may decide to do the fFN test to see if there is a risk for premature delivery.
- There is a lower risk of preterm birth when the test result for fFN is negative after 22 weeks and before 35 weeks of pregnancy.
- A swab of cervical-vaginal secretions is taken from the top of the vagina, behind the cervix, then sent to the lab, where it is tested for fFN.
- Results are available within 24 hours.
- If fFN is present after 22 weeks, it indicates increased risk for preterm delivery.
- If it is absent, the risk is low, and the woman probably won't deliver in the next 2 weeks.

Treatment of Premature Labor

- We can now treat premature labor in several different ways.

- The treatment most often used for premature labor is *bed rest.* A woman is advised to stay in bed and lie on her side.
- Not everyone agrees on this treatment, but bed rest is often successful in stopping contractions and premature labor.
- If this happens to you and you are advised to rest in bed, it may mean you can't go to work or to continue many activities.
- It's worth it to agree to bed rest if you can avoid premature delivery of your baby.
- If you are confined to bed during your pregnancy, be careful resuming activities and getting back into the swing of things after baby is born.
- Lying down for quite a while may result in loss of muscle tone, which can lead to you being out of shape. It can take time to return to your normal level of activity after extended bed rest.
- Take it easy, and don't rush into any physical activities until you feel up to them. Ease into your post-bed-rest life slowly!

Medications to Help Stop Premature Labor

- Beta-adrenergic agents, also called *tocolytic agents,* may be used to suppress labor.

- Beta-adrenergics are muscle relaxants. They relax the uterus and decrease contractions. (The uterus is mainly muscle; it is the tightening or contraction of the uterus that pushes the baby out through the cervix during labor.)
- At this time, only *ritodrine (Yutopar)* is approved by the FDA to treat premature labor.
- Ritodrine is approved for use between 20 and 36 weeks of pregnancy.
- Ritodrine is given in three different forms—intravenously, as an intramuscular injection and as a pill.
- In some cases, the medication is used in women with a history of premature labor or for a woman with multiple pregnancies.
- It is usually initially given intravenously and may require a hospital stay of a couple of days or more.
- When premature contractions stop, you may be switched to oral medications, which you take every 2 to 4 hours.
- *Terbutaline* may also be used as a muscle relaxant to halt premature labor.
- Although it has been shown to be an effective medication and is used frequently for this purpose, it has not been approved for this use by the FDA.
- *Magnesium sulfate* is used to treat pre-eclampsia; we have known for quite a while that magnesium sulfate may also help stop premature labor.

- You must be monitored frequently if you take magnesium sulfate.
- *Sedatives* or *narcotics* may also be used in early attempts to stop labor; this may be an injection of morphine or meperidine (Demerol).
- It is not a long-term solution but may be effective in initially stopping labor.
- A recent study showed that use of the hormone *progesterone (17 alpha-hydroxyprogesterone caproate)* in some women may reduce their risk of giving birth to a premature baby.
- In the study, women who had had problems with premature labor in previous pregnancies were given a weekly injection of progesterone.
- This course of treatment substantially reduced the rate of premature deliveries. More studies are needed, but there is hope that this treatment will lead to a decrease in premature birth, which can be a very serious problem.

Benefits of Stopping Premature Labor

- Benefits of stopping premature labor include reducing the risks of fetal problems and problems related to premature delivery.
- If you experience premature labor, you may need to see your doctor more frequently.

- Your doctor will probably monitor your pregnancy with ultrasound, nonstress tests, contraction-stress tests and biophysical profiles.

Home Uterine Monitoring

- Some women are monitored at home during pregnancy with home uterine monitoring.
- Contractions of a pregnant woman's uterus are recorded once or more during the day, then transmitted by telephone to the doctor or a nurse for evaluation.
- The procedure is used to identify women at risk of premature labor.
- Costs vary but run between $80 and $100 a day.

Some Late-Pregnancy Problems

What Is Pre-eclampsia?

Pre-eclampsia describes a variety of symptoms that occur only during pregnancy or shortly after delivery.

- Symptoms of pre-eclampsia include swelling (edema), protein in the urine (proteinuria), hypertension (high blood pressure) and a change in reflexes (hyperreflexia).

- Other nonspecific, important symptoms of pre-eclampsia include pain under the ribs on the right side, headache, seeing spots or other changes in vision.
- These are all warning signs. Report them to your doctor immediately, particularly if you've had blood-pressure problems during pregnancy!
- Most pregnant women have some swelling during pregnancy; swelling in the legs does *not* mean you have pre-eclampsia.
- It is also possible to have hypertension during pregnancy without having pre-eclampsia.
- Laboratory tests include *h*emolysis, *e*levated *l*iver enzymes and *l*ow *p*latelet counts (HELLP syndrome).
- HELLP syndrome is severe pre-eclampsia and is associated with increased risks for mother and fetus.
- We are not certain what causes pre-eclampsia, but one study showed that women who developed pre-eclampsia had a specific protein present in the cells of their placenta. This protein binds two growth factors that are needed for healthy fetal development. A great deal more research needs to be done, but we may be on the right track to understanding and treating this pregnancy problem in the future.
- Pre-eclampsia occurs most often during a woman's first pregnancy.

- Other risk factors include carrying more than one baby, pre-eclampsia in a previous pregnancy, chronic high blood pressure, diabetes, obesity, being older and being African-American.
- Women over 30 years old who are having their first baby are more likely to develop high blood pressure and pre-eclampsia.
- Some researchers believe that working women are more likely to develop pre-eclampsia due to *job stress.*
- If you are in a stressful job situation, discuss it with your physician.
- Other researchers believe the tendency to develop the problem is genetically inherited.
- The goal in treating pre-eclampsia is to avoid eclampsia (seizures). See the explanation below.
- Weight gain can be a sign of pre-eclampsia or worsening pre-eclampsia, due to increased water retention.
- Treatment of pre-eclampsia begins with bed rest at home. You may not be able to work or to spend much time on your feet.
- Bed rest allows for the most efficient functioning of your kidneys and the greatest blood flow to the uterus.
- Lie on your side, not on your back.
- Drink lots of water.
- Avoid salt, salty foods and foods that contain sodium, which may make you retain fluid.

- If you can't rest at home in bed or if symptoms do not improve, you may be admitted to the hospital or your baby may need to be delivered.
- A baby is delivered to avoid seizures in you and for the baby's well-being.
- During labor, pre-eclampsia may be treated with magnesium sulfate. It is given by I.V. to prevent seizures during and after delivery.
- Pre-eclampsia can progress to *eclampsia*. Eclampsia refers to seizures or convulsions in a woman with pre-eclampsia.
- Seizures are not caused by a previous history of epilepsy or a seizure disorder.
- If you think you've had a seizure, call your doctor immediately!
- Eclampsia is treated with medications similar to those prescribed for seizure disorders.

Tips for the Expectant Dad

What Can I Do? How Can I Help?

If your partner has any problems during her pregnancy, be supportive of her. She's probably scared about what is happening—you may be, too—so work together to reassure each other. Times like these help you develop a closeness and bond that will benefit you as you begin your life as a family.

Placental Abruption

- Placental abruption is premature separation of the placenta from the wall of the uterus.
- Normally, the placenta does not separate from the uterus until after the baby is delivered.
- Separation before delivery can be very serious.
- Placental abruption occurs in about 1 in every 200 deliveries. The cause of placental abruption is unknown.
- Certain conditions may increase the chance of placental abruption, including:
  ~ physical injury to the mother, as from a car accident
  ~ a short umbilical cord
  ~ sudden change in the size of the uterus (from delivery or rupture of membranes)
  ~ hypertension
  ~ dietary deficiency
  ~ a uterine abnormality, such as a band of tissue in the uterus where the placenta cannot attach properly
  ~ previous surgery on the uterus (removal of fibroids) or D&C for abortion or miscarriage
  ~ pre-eclampsia
  ~ uterine fibroids
  ~ increased maternal age and a higher number of pregnancies
  ~ cocaine use

- Folic-acid deficiency may play a role in causing placental abruption.
- Mothers who smoke and drink alcohol during pregnancy may be more likely to have placental abruption.
- A woman who has had placental abruption in the past is at increased risk of having it recur. Rate of recurrence has been estimated to be as high as 10%.
- Separation of the placenta may involve partial or total separation from the uterine wall.
- The situation is most severe when the placenta separates totally from the uterine wall.
- The baby relies entirely on circulation from the placenta. When it separates, the baby cannot receive blood from the umbilical cord, which is attached to the placenta.
- Symptoms of placental abruption can vary a great deal. There may be heavy bleeding from the vagina, or you may experience no bleeding at all.
- Other symptoms can include lower-back pain, tenderness of the uterus or abdomen, and contractions or tightening of the uterus.
- Ultrasound may be helpful in diagnosing this problem, although it does not always provide an exact diagnosis.
- Serious problems, such as shock due to the rapid loss of large quantities of blood, may occur with premature separation of the placenta.

- Blood clotting can also be a problem.
- Treatment of placental abruption varies.
  - ~ With heavy bleeding, delivery of the baby may be necessary.
  - ~ When bleeding is not heavy, the problem may be treated with a more conservative approach. This depends on whether the fetus is in distress or in immediate danger.
- Placental abruption is one of the most serious problems related to the 2nd and 3rd trimesters of pregnancy. If you have any symptoms, call your doctor immediately!

Placenta Previa

With *placenta previa*, the placenta lies close to the cervix or covers the cervix; it happens about once in every 170 pregnancies. Placenta previa is serious because of the chance of heavy bleeding. Bleeding may occur during pregnancy or during labor.

- Risk factors for an increased chance of placenta previa include previous Cesarean delivery, many pregnancies and a mother who is older.
- Smoking also increases the risk of placenta previa.
- The most characteristic symptom of placenta previa is painless bleeding without any contractions of the uterus.

- Bleeding with placenta previa doesn't usually occur until close to the end of your 2nd trimester or later when the cervix thins out, stretches and tears the placenta loose.
- Bleeding with placenta previa may occur without warning and may be extremely heavy. It occurs when the cervix begins to dilate with early labor, and blood escapes.
- The problem cannot be diagnosed with an exam because a pelvic examination may cause heavier bleeding.
- Doctors use ultrasound to identify placenta previa. Ultrasound is particularly accurate in the second half of pregnancy as the uterus and placenta get bigger.
- If you have placenta previa, your doctor may tell you not to have a pelvic exam. This is important to remember if you see another doctor or when you go to the hospital.
- The baby is more likely to be in a breech position with placenta previa. For this reason, and to control bleeding, a Cesarean delivery is usually performed.
- Cesarean delivery allows the doctor to deliver the baby, then remove the placenta so the uterus can contract. Bleeding can be kept to a minimum.
- It is not possible to deliver the placenta safely before the baby.

Vasa Previa

- *Vasa previa* is a condition in which blood vessels from the umbilical cord cross the interior opening of the cervix, lying close to it or covering it.
- These blood vessels can rupture due to the pressure and tearing caused when the cervix dilates; this can cause serious bleeding.
- The condition is also associated with a high rate of fetal death.
- The danger to the fetus with vasa previa is that with rupture of the membranes, fetal vessels may also rupture, causing blood loss from the fetus.
- Vasa previa occurs in about 1 in 3000 pregnancies.

Tips for the Expectant Dad
What Can I Do? How Can I Help?

Make sure your partner knows how to find you and/or how to get in touch with you now. Then she won't worry about getting to the hospital or fret about problems she may experience, such as bleeding or her water breaking. Keep your cell phone handy, if you have one, or carry a pager. Make sure she has phone numbers where she can reach you.

Part II: As Your Labor Begins

What Is Labor?

- Labor is the occurrence of uterine contractions sufficient to cause stretching and dilatation of your cervix, which is the opening of the uterus.
- The cervix opens while your uterus, which is a muscle, tightens to push out your baby.
- When you are in labor, this tightening (contraction) can cause pain.
- During labor, your bladder, rectum, spine and pubic bone receive strong pressure from the uterus as it tightens and hardens with each contraction. This usually causes pain.
- The weight of the baby's head as it moves down the birth canal also causes pressure or pain.
- Labor is different for every woman, so no one can predict what your labor will be like before it begins.
- Labor may feel like cramps for some women.
- For others, their back might hurt.
- No two labors are alike, not even for the same woman.
- Some women experience long, intense labors; others have short, relatively pain-free labors.

- Labor is divided into three stages—each stage feels distinctly different and has a specific purpose. See the discussion below.
- You may bleed a small amount following a vaginal exam late in pregnancy or at the beginning of labor.
- This is called a *bloody show* and occurs as the cervix stretches and dilates.
- Along with light bleeding, you may pass some mucus, called a *mucus plug.*
- During labor, you won't be allowed to eat or to drink anything.
- Women often get nauseated during labor, which could cause vomiting.
- You may be able to sip water or to suck on ice chips.

What Is Back Labor?

- Some women experience back labor; it occurs in about 30% of all deliveries.
- *Back labor* means most of the pain is concentrated in the lower back.
- Back labor may be caused by your baby facing toward your front (posterior position).
- During labor, it's better if the baby is looking down at the ground so it can extend its head as it comes out through the birth canal.

- If the baby can't extend its head, its chin points toward its chest. This can cause pain in your lower back.
- Each contraction forces the baby's head against your lower spine, resulting in strong pain that may not completely disappear between contractions.
- With back labor, labor and delivery may take longer.
- The doctor may have to rotate the baby's head so it comes out looking down at the ground rather than up at the sky.

Tips for the Expectant Dad *What Can I Do? How Can I Help?*

Labor is the time to use what you learned in your prenatal classes—it can really pay off. If you learned breathing methods to ease tension or pain, do them now. Massage your partner's sore or tense spots, if she wants you to. Help her walk around. Tell her you love her and are excited about what is happening.

Dealing with Labor Pain before You Go to the Hospital

If you're waiting to go to the hospital and are experiencing pain, there are a few things you can do at home. The following actions may help you manage your pain.

- At the beginning of each contraction, take a deep breath, then let it out slowly. At the end of the contraction, again breathe deeply.

- Get up and move! It helps distract you and may relieve back pain.
- Ask your partner to massage your shoulders, neck, back and feet. Massage helps ease tension, and it feels good.
- Hot and/or cold compresses can help reduce cramping and various aches and pains. A warm shower or bath can also feel very good.
- When a contraction begins, try to distract yourself with mental pictures of pleasant or soothing images.

Timing Contractions

- Contractions are caused by your uterus tightening and relaxing during labor to expel the baby.
- It's important for your doctor to know how often contractions occur and how long each one lasts. Timing contractions provides this information.
- Ask your doctor how he or she prefers you to time your contractions.
- There are two ways to do it.
  - ~ *Method 1.* Start timing when the contraction starts, and time it until the next contraction starts. This is the most common method.
  - ~ *Method 2.* Start timing when the contraction ends, and note how long it is until the next contraction starts.

Tips for the Expectant Dad *What Can I Do? How Can I Help?*

Know how to time your partner's contractions, and help her in this important task. Timing contractions provides your doctor with information to help him or her decide whether it's time for you both to go to the hospital, and it gives you something to do to pass the time.

Three Stages of Labor

- There are three distinct stages of labor:
  - ~ **Stage one**—The first stage of labor begins with uterine contractions of great enough intensity, duration and frequency to cause the cervix to thin (effacement) and open (dilatation). The first stage of labor ends when the cervix is fully dilated (10cm) and sufficiently open to allow the baby's head to come through it.
  - ~ **Stage two**—The second stage of labor begins when the cervix is completely dilated at 10cm. This stage ends with the delivery of the baby.
  - ~ **Stage three**—The third stage of labor begins after delivery of the baby. It ends with delivery of the placenta and the membranes that have surrounded the fetus.
- Some doctors have even described a fourth stage of labor, referring to a time period after delivery of the placenta during which the uterus contracts.

- Contraction of the uterus is important in controlling bleeding that can occur after delivery of the baby and placenta. See the discussion of bleeding after delivery on page 139.

How Long Will Labor Last?

- The length of the first and second stages of labor, from the beginning of cervical dilatation to delivery of the baby, can last 14 to 15 hours or more in a first pregnancy.
- Women have had faster labors than this, but don't count on it.
- A woman who has already had one or two children will probably have a shorter labor, but don't count on that either!
- The average time for labor is usually decreased by a few hours for a second or third delivery.
- Everyone's heard of women who barely made it to the hospital or had a 1-hour labor. For every one of those patients, there are many women who have labored 18, 20, 24 hours or longer.
- It's almost impossible to predict the amount of time that will be required for labor. You may ask your doctor about it, but his or her answer is only a guess.

Tips for the Expectant Dad *What Can I Do? How Can I Help?*

At the hospital, offer to make phone calls for your partner. She may want you to call to excuse her from work or to call family members and friends to let them know her labor has started.

Your Partner Is Important

- Before your delivery date, talk with your partner about how you will stay in touch as your due date approaches.
- Some people rent personal pagers for the last few weeks. (Some hospitals and health-maintenance organizations supply pagers for expectant couples.)
- If you have a cellular phone, staying in touch is fairly easy.
- You may be able to borrow a cell phone from a friend or family member if you don't have one.
- Arrange for a backup support person, in case your partner cannot be with you or you need someone else to take you to the hospital.
- Your partner can help prepare you for labor and delivery, and support you as you labor.
- He can share the joy of your baby's delivery with you.

- He can support you emotionally, which is very important to you both.
- Your partner may choose to be your labor coach.
- You may want your partner to videotape or photograph the birth.
- On the other hand, you may *not* want him to do this. Talk with him about it.

When Your Water Breaks

- As your labor begins, the membranes that surround the baby and hold the fluid ("bag of waters") may break, and fluid leaks from your vagina.
- You may feel a gush of fluid, followed by slow leaking, or you may just feel a slow leaking, without the gush of fluid.
- A *continuous* leakage of fluid is a good clue that your water has broken.
- A sanitary pad helps absorb any leaking amniotic fluid.
- Amniotic fluid is usually clear and watery. Occasionally it may have a bloody appearance, or it may be yellow or green.
- Not every woman's water breaks before labor begins. Often membranes rupture during labor, or the

physician ruptures the membranes when you are in labor.

- Occasionally the bag of waters breaks prematurely, before baby is ready to be born.
- There are several ways a doctor can confirm if your membranes have ruptured.
  - ~ *By your description of what happened.* For example, if you describe a large gush of fluid from your vagina.
  - ~ *With nitrazine paper.* Fluid is placed on the paper; if membranes have ruptured, the paper changes color.
  - ~ *With a ferning test.* Fluid from the vagina is placed on a glass slide, allowed to dry, then examined under a microscope. A fernlike appearance indicates it is amniotic fluid.

What Do You Do When Your Water Breaks?

- Your membranes may rupture at any point in pregnancy. Don't assume it will happen only around the time of labor.
- If you believe your water has broken, call your doctor immediately.
- Avoid sexual intercourse if you think your water has broken. Intercourse can increase the possibility of

introducing an infection into your uterus and thus to your baby.

- The risk of infection increases when your water breaks.

Lightening—Will Your Baby Drop?

- A few weeks before labor begins or at the beginning of labor, you may notice a change in your abdomen.
- When your doctor examines you, the measurement from your bellybutton or the pubic symphysis to the top of the uterus may be smaller than what you noticed on a previous visit.
- This phenomenon occurs as the head of the baby enters the birth canal; it is often called *lightening*.
- Pregnant women often describe the feeling by saying, "The baby has dropped."
- Don't be concerned if you don't notice lightening or a drop of the fetus. It doesn't occur with every woman or with every pregnancy.
- It's also common for your baby to drop just before labor begins or during labor.
- With lightening, you may experience benefits and problems.

- One benefit may be more room in your upper abdomen. This gives you more room to breathe because there's room for your lungs to expand.
- However, with the descent of the baby, you may notice pressure in your pelvis, bladder and rectum, which can make you uncomfortable.
- In some instances, your doctor may examine you and tell you your baby is "not in the pelvis" or "is high up."
- He or she is saying the baby has not yet descended into the birth canal, but this situation can change quickly.
- If your doctor says your baby is "floating" or "ballotable," it means part of the baby is felt high in the birth canal. But the baby is not engaged (fixed) in the birth canal at this point. The baby may even move away from your doctor's fingers when you are examined.

The Baby's Birth Position
(Presentation)

Most babies enter the birth canal head first, which is the best position for labor and delivery. Some babies enter the birth canal in other presentations. There is a difference between birth *presentation* and birth *position*. *Presentation* refers to the part of the baby that enters the birth canal first. *Position* refers to the relation of a part of the baby to the right or left side of the birth canal.

- Breech presentation occurs in 3 to 4% of term pregnancies.
- A *breech presentation* means the baby is not in a head-down position; its legs or buttocks come into the birth canal first.
- If your baby is breech when it is time to deliver, your doctor may try to turn the baby or you may need a Cesarean delivery.
- One of the main causes of a breech presentation is prematurity of the baby. Near the end of the 2nd trimester, the baby is commonly in the breech presentation. As you move through the 3rd trimester, the baby usually turns into the head-down presentation for birth.
- For a long time, breech deliveries were vaginal.
- Then doctors believed it was safer to do a C-section for a breech baby. Many still do so today.
- Some physicians believe you can deliver a breech baby vaginally, without difficulty, if the situation is right.

- There are other presentations that are not normal; they include the following.
    - ~ A *Frank breech occurs* when baby's legs are straight and bent at the hips so it is in a jack-knife position. Feet are up by the face or head.
    - ~ In a *complete breech presentation,* one or both knees are bent.
    - ~ With an *incomplete breech presentation,* a foot or knee enters the birth canal ahead of the rest of the baby.
    - ~ In a *face presentation,* the baby's head is hyper-extended so the face enters the birth canal first.
    - ~ If baby is in a *transverse lie,* it is lying almost as if in a cradle in your pelvis. The head is on one side of your abdomen, and the bottom is on the other side.
    - ~ With a *shoulder presentation,* the baby's shoulder enters the birth canal first.

Tips for the Expectant Dad
What Can I Do? How Can I Help?

It might be fun for both of you if your partner asks the doctor to draw baby's position on her tummy with a marker at one of her exams to show how the baby is lying at that time.

Turning Your Baby

- If your baby is breech, your doctor may try to change its presentation by using a technique called *external cephalic version (ECV)* or just *version*.
- An ultrasound is usually done first so the doctor can see the presentation of the baby and again during the procedure to guide the doctor in changing baby's presentation.
- Tocolytics (medication to prevent contractions or labor) are often given at the same time ECV is attempted.
- The doctor places his or her hands on your abdomen. Using gentle pressure on your uterus, he or she tries to shift the baby into the head-down presentation.
- The gentle pressure causes the baby to do a somersault to change to the head-down presentation (vertex).
- This method is usually used before your water breaks and before labor begins.
- ECV is not usually done until at least 36 weeks of pregnancy.
- It is successful in about half of the cases in which it is used.
- Not every doctor is trained in the procedure.
- A doctor may be successful in turning the baby; however, some stubborn babies shift again into a breech presentation after they are turned.

- ECV may be tried once more, but version is harder to perform as your delivery date draws closer.
- Problems can occur with ECV; discuss the situation with your doctor.
- One new technique to turn baby (at least new here in the U.S.) that is being used is *moxibustion.*
- It is a form of ancient Chinese therapy in which bundles of specific herbs are burned near the little (outside) toes on a woman's feet.
- This is done every day for 1 to 2 weeks.
- It may sound weird, but it works, and with no danger to the mom or baby!
- For further information on moxibustion, contact NCCAOM at 888-330-6222.

Delivering a Breech Baby

- For many years, most breech deliveries were performed vaginally. Then it was believed the safest method was C-section, especially if it was a first baby.
- Many doctors today believe a Cesarean section is still the safest method of delivering a breech baby.
- Ask your doctor what he or she normally does in this situation.

- If your baby is breech, tell the nurses when you get to the hospital.
- If you call with a question about labor and have a breech presentation, mention this information to the person you talk with.
- ACOG (the American College of Obstetricians and Gynecologists) recommends ECV when possible.
- However, they also recommend that a persistent breech presentation (the baby won't move or moves back into a breech presentation after ECV) at term should be delivered by C-section.

Preparing to Go to the Hospital

- You may want to preregister at the hospital a few weeks before your due date to save time checking in when you are actually in labor.
- Preregistration forms are available from your doctor's office or the hospital.
- Fill out the forms early.
- Take your insurance card or insurance information with you—put it on top of the things you pack in your bag.
- Know your blood type and Rh-factor, your doctor's name, your pediatrician's name and your due date.

- At one of your prenatal visits, ask your physician the following questions.
    - ~ When should I go to the hospital once I am in labor?
    - ~ Should I call you before I leave for the hospital?
    - ~ How can I reach you after regular office hours?
    - ~ Are there any particular instructions to follow during early labor?
- Going to the hospital to have a baby can make anyone a little nervous, so make some plans before you go and you'll have less to worry about.
    - ~ Tour the labor and delivery area of your hospital with your partner.
    - ~ Preregister at the hospital.
    - ~ Talk to your doctor about what will happen during your labor.
    - ~ Find out who might cover for your doctor if he or she cannot be there for the birth.
    - ~ Plan the trip, and drive it with your partner a couple of times.
    - ~ Make alternative plans in case your partner cannot be with you.
    - ~ Know how to get in touch with your partner 24 hours a day.
    - ~ Pack your bag with items for you, your labor coach or partner, and the baby.

- If you are unsure about whether it's time to go to the hospital, don't be afraid to call your doctor or the hospital.
- General guidelines for going to the hospital include:
  ~ you believe your water has broken
  ~ you are bleeding
  ~ you have contractions every 5 minutes, lasting 1 minute

Tips for the Expectant Dad *What Can I Do? How Can I Help?*

If your partner asks you to make phone calls for her to the doctor or the hospital, do it. She may be in pain, or she may be scared. Helping her in this way shows you are supporting her.

At the Hospital

The Labor Check

If you think you may be in labor and go to the hospital, you will have a labor check.

- A labor check is usually done in labor and delivery.
- Vital signs will be taken, a monitor will be placed on your abdomen and a pelvic exam will be performed.
- The monitor checks your contractions and baby's heartbeat.

- These tests are done to determine if you are in labor and if your pregnancy is doing OK.
- If you are not in labor, you will be given instructions and sent home.
- Your instructions usually include precautions and warning signs.
- No one wants to be sent home, but it is OK. You'll be back soon.

Once You're Admitted

- Once you're admitted to the hospital, many things happen.
- A copy of your office chart is usually kept on record in labor and delivery. It contains basic information about your health and pregnancy.
- However, you will probably be asked many questions when you check in. They may include the following.
  - ~ Have your membranes ruptured? At what time?
  - ~ Are you bleeding?
  - ~ Are you having contractions? How often do they occur? How long do they last?
  - ~ When did you last eat and what did you eat?
- Other important information for you to share includes medical problems you have and any medications you take or have taken during pregnancy.

- If you've had complications during this pregnancy, such as placenta previa, tell medical personnel when you first come to labor and delivery.
- This is also the time to tell those taking care of you any information your doctor gave you at your last exam about effacement, dilatation of the cervix and station.

Tips for the Expectant Dad
What Can I Do? How Can I Help?

Offer to answer the phone in the labor room. It's a good idea to screen calls from anxious and inquisitive family and friends. Or turn off the phone if you don't want to be disturbed.

Your Initial Exam

- A pelvic exam is performed to help determine what stage of labor you are in and to use as a reference point for future exams during labor.
- This exam and the vital signs are done by a labor-and-delivery nurse (the nurse can be male or female).
- You will be checked to see how much your cervix has dilated and to make sure baby's head is coming first.
- A brief history of your pregnancy is taken.
- Your blood pressure, pulse and temperature are taken, and your baby's heart rate is noted.

- Blood will probably be drawn.
- You may have an intravenous (I.V.) drip started in your arm. It is necessary with an epidural anesthesia; however, if you have chosen not to have an epidural, an I.V. is not always required. Ask your doctor about it at a prenatal appointment.
- An I.V. is a good safety precaution for problems; medications and/or blood can be administered quickly.
- Most physicians agree an I.V. is also helpful if a woman needs fluids during labor.
- You may have an epidural put in place, if you request one.
- Only in unusual situations, such as in an emergency, will your doctor do the initial exam.
- In fact, it may be quite awhile before you see your doctor, but rest assured the nurses are in close telephone contact with him or her.
- In many labors, the doctor does not arrive until close to delivery.

Will You Have an Enema?

- Some women are concerned about having an enema during their labor.

- An *enema* is a procedure in which fluid is injected into the rectum for the purpose of clearing out the bowel.
- Most hospitals offer an enema at the beginning of labor, but it is not always mandatory.
- There are certain advantages to having an enema early in labor.
  - ~ An enema before labor or at the beginning of labor can make the birth of your baby a more pleasant experience.
  - ~ When the baby's head comes out through the birth canal, anything in the rectum comes out, too.
  - ~ An enema decreases the amount of contamination by bowel movement or feces during labor and at the time of delivery, preventing possible infection.
  - ~ You may not want to have a bowel movement soon after your baby's birth because of discomfort with an episiotomy.
  - ~ Having an enema before labor can prevent this discomfort.
- Ask your doctor if an enema is routine or considered helpful.
- Tell him or her you'd like to know about the benefits of an enema and the reason for giving one.
- It isn't required by all doctors or all hospitals.

Will You Need to Be Shaved?

- Many women want to know if they have to have their pubic hair shaved before the birth of their baby. It is not a requirement any longer; many women are not shaved these days.

- Some women who chose not to have their pubic hair shaved later said they experienced discomfort when their pubic hair became entangled in their underwear due to the normal vaginal discharge after the birth of their baby.

- Usually the area around the vagina (perineum) is washed or scrubbed with a sponge and soap or betadine.

- If there is hair in the area, it can be trimmed with scissors or a minishave prep can be done.

- You might want to think about this procedure, and discuss it with your doctor at a prenatal visit.

When Your Doctor Isn't Available

- In some cases, when you get to the hospital you'll learn your doctor is not available, and someone else will deliver your baby.

- If your doctor believes he or she might be out of town when your baby is born, ask who "covers" when your doctor is unavailable.

- Ask to schedule a prenatal visit with doctors that cover for your doctor.
- Although your physician would like to be there for the birth of your baby, sometimes it is not possible.

Tips for the Expectant Dad *What Can I Do? How Can I Help?*

Be in charge of the door or curtain to the labor room. Your partner may be stuck in bed, and there will be times she won't want the door opened or people entering the room, such as during a pelvic exam or if she receives an enema.

Tests for You and Your Baby

You may wonder how your doctor can tell your baby is all right, especially during labor.

- In many hospitals, the baby's heart rate is monitored throughout labor so problems can be detected early and resolved.
- Labor can be stressful for a baby.
- Every time the uterus contracts during labor, less oxygenated blood flows from you to the placenta.
- Most babies can handle this stress without any problem.
- When a baby cannot handle the stress, it is called *fetal stress*.

Fetal Monitoring
(Electronic Fetal Monitoring)

- In many hospitals, a baby's heartbeat is monitored throughout labor with external fetal monitoring or internal fetal monitoring.

- A normal fetal heart rate ranges from 110 to 160 beats a minute.

- There are two ways to monitor the baby's heartbeat during labor—*internal* and *external fetal monitoring*.

- *External fetal monitoring* can be done before your membranes rupture.

- A pair of belts are strapped to your abdomen to record your contractions and the baby's heartbeat.

- One strap holds an ultrasound to monitor fetal heart rate. The other strap holds a device to measure the length of contractions and how often they occur.

- *Internal fetal monitoring* monitors the baby and your contractions more precisely.

- Only women whose membranes are broken and who are dilated at least 1cm can be attached to an internal fetal monitor.

- An electrode, called a *scalp electrode,* is placed through the vagina and cervix, then attached to the fetus's scalp. The electrode is connected by wires to a machine that records the fetal heart rate.

- A thin tube, called an *internal uterine pressure catheter*, can be put inside the uterus to monitor the frequency, intensity and duration of contractions.
- It may be a little uncomfortable to have monitors placed or inserted, but it is not painful.
- Monitors send information to a machine that records the information on a strip of paper.
- Monitor results can usually be seen in your room and at the nurses' station. In some places, your doctor can check results on his or her computer.
- In most cases, when you are monitored, you must stay in bed. In some places, wireless monitors are available so you can move around.

Tips for the Expectant Dad
What Can I Do? How Can I Help?

You and your partner should discuss ahead of time her feelings and your feelings about certain treatments, so you can be supportive of her when it's time to make decisions. During labor, there may be things you and your partner want to discuss alone. It may be helpful to arrange ahead of time a signal that lets the other know you want to talk privately.

Fetal Blood Sampling

- Your doctor can test your baby's blood pH to see how well your baby is tolerating the stress of labor.

- Before this test can be done, your membranes must be ruptured, and you must be dilated at least 2cm.
- An instrument makes a small nick in baby's scalp.
- Baby's blood is collected in a small tube, and its pH (acidity) is checked.
- If the baby is having trouble with labor and is under stress, the pH level can help determine this.
- This test can help your doctor decide whether labor can continue or if a C-section needs to be done.

A Test for Baby's Oxygen Level

- We can now monitor baby's oxygen *inside* the womb, before birth.
- This test is not available everywhere.
- Light measures the oxygen level in fetal blood, providing an accurate answer as to whether baby's oxygen levels are in the safe range.
- This test, called *OxiFirst* fetal oxygen monitoring, is used during labor.
- Studies have shown the test increases the effectiveness of fetal-heart monitors.
- If an abnormal heart rate is found—this occurs in 30% of all births in which monitors are used—oxygen levels can be helpful in determining whether a C-section should be performed.

- A sensor is passed through the birth canal and placed on the baby's cheek, where it measures the oxygen with a harmless infrared light.
- If low oxygen levels are detected, decisions can be made about delivering the baby.

Laboring Positions

- Most women in North America and Europe give birth on their backs, in bed.
- Although lying on your back is the most common position used for labor, it can decrease the strength and frequency of contractions, which can slow the labor process.
- It can also make your blood pressure drop and cause your baby's heart rate to drop, particularly if you are flat on your back.
- If you lie on your back, elevate the head of the bed and put a pillow under one hip so you are not lying flat.
- Some women try different positions to find relief from pain and to make the birth of their baby easier.
- In the past, women often labored and gave birth in an upright position, such as kneeling, squatting, sitting or standing up; these positions kept the pelvis vertical.

- Laboring in these positions may enable the abdominal wall to relax and the baby to descend more rapidly.
- Because contractions are stronger and more regular, labor is often shorter.
- Today, many women are asking to choose the labor and birth position that is most comfortable for them.
- Freedom to choose the labor and birth position can make you feel more confident about managing birth and labor.
- If this is important to you, discuss the matter with your doctor.
- Ask about the facilities at the hospital you will use; some have special equipment, such as birthing chairs, squatting bars or birthing beds, to help you feel more comfortable.
- Positions you might consider for your labor are described below.
- *Walking* and *standing* are good positions to use during early labor.
- Walking may help you breathe more easily and help you relax more.
- When walking, be sure someone is with you to offer support (both physical and emotional).
- Some women want to know if walking during labor makes labor easier and reduces the chance of a C-section.

- A recent study found that walking did not provide any harm *or* benefit over resting in bed. Walking together can help pass the time for you and your partner.
- The study concluded a woman should be allowed to choose whichever option works best for her.
- Standing in a warm shower may provide relief.
- *Sitting* can decrease the strength and frequency of contractions and can slow labor.
- Sitting to rest after walking or standing is acceptable; however, sitting can be uncomfortable during a contraction.
- *Kneeling on hands and knees* is a good way to relieve the pain of back labor.
- *Kneeling against a support,* such as a chair or your partner, stretches your back muscles.
- The effects of kneeling are similar to those of walking and standing.
- When you can't stand, walk or kneel, *lie on your side.*
- If you receive pain medication, you will need to lie down. Lie on your left side, then turn to your right.
- Discuss the situation with your labor nurse, who can help you find comfortable positions for you that are also beneficial for your baby.

Tips for the Expectant Dad
What Can I Do? How Can I Help?

Some of the different laboring positions require your assistance. Help your partner by letting her lean on you or supporting her in various ways, such as with your arm around her or walking behind her to make sure she doesn't fall.

Coping with the Pain of Labor and Childbirth

Childbirth is usually accompanied by pain. The amount varies among women, from very little to a great deal. The best way to deal with pain is to become informed about it. Many women (or their partners) believe they should not ask for pain relief during labor.

- Some women think the baby will be harmed by any medication used during labor and/or delivery.
- Other women believe they'll deprive themselves of the "complete birth experience" if they receive pain medication.
- A few women are concerned about cost and believe they can't afford an epidural if their insurance doesn't cover it.

- Learn about pain and pain-relief methods so you'll be informed.
- Childbirth-education classes are good sources of information.
- You can learn about pain-relief methods that don't require medication, such as breathing methods and relaxation techniques.
- Discuss pain relief with your doctor at a prenatal visit. And discuss it with your partner *before* labor begins.
- Keep an open mind about using medication for pain relief during labor—your labor may be harder (or easier) than you expect.
- Using medication for pain relief is usually a personal choice, not a medical decision, except in the case of a Cesarean delivery.
- You can always change your mind if you need to or want to.

Tips for the Expectant Dad
What Can I Do? How Can I Help?

Be a positive influence during labor and delivery—keep a positive attitude. Labor and delivery can be a scary process for both of you, but it helps if you concentrate on the miracle you are sharing.

Pain Relief without Medication

- Some women do not want to use medication during labor to relieve pain.
- They prefer to use different laboring positions, massage, breathing patterns, relaxation techniques or hypnotherapy to relieve their discomfort.
- Breathing patterns and relaxation techniques are usually learned in childbirth-education classes.
- Some women are now trying different labor positions to find relief from pain and to make the birth of their baby easier. See the discussion that begins on page 86.
- If a different laboring position is important to you, talk to your doctor about it.
- In some places, *hypnosis* to relieve pain during childbirth is used by some women.
- *HypnoBirthing* is a labor-pain management technique developed by Marie Mongan over 20 years ago.
- Ask your doctor about it at one of your prenatal visits if you are interested.
- Classes may be available in your area.
- *Aromatherapy* consists of massage with certain aromatic oils.
- It can be helpful for relaxation during labor.
- *Birth pools* may be available in some hospitals.

- Some women experience a reduction in pain and an increase in relaxation when they are in the water.
- The water also softens the perineal area, so it may stretch more easily.
- In most hospitals, you have to get out of the pool to give birth.
- Discuss it with your doctor if you are interested.
- *Acupressure* uses pressure on areas of the body to help relieve pain and to relax you.
- It may also give you a sense of well-being.
- For acupressure to work most effectively, it must usually be started at the beginning of labor. Ask your doctor about it if you are interested.

Massage for Relief

- The touching and caressing of massage may help you relax during labor.
- Many parts of the body of a laboring woman can be massaged.
- Massaging the head, neck, back and feet can offer a great deal of comfort and relaxation.
- The person doing the massage should pay close attention to your responses to determine correct pressure.
- *Effleurage* is light, gentle fingertip massage over the abdomen and upper thighs; it is used during early

labor. Stroking is light, but doesn't tickle, and fingertips never leave the skin.

- Your partner or labor coach can begin with hands on either side of the navel. Hands move upward and outward, and come back down to the pubic area. Then they move back up to the navel.
- Massage may extend down the thighs.
- It can also be done as a crosswise motion, around fetal-monitor belts.
- Fingers are moved across the abdomen from one side to the other, between the belts.
- *Counterpressure massage* is excellent for relieving the pain of back labor.
- The heel of the hand or the flat part of the fist of the person giving the massage should be placed against the tailbone.
- Firm pressure is applied in a small, circular motion.
- A tennis ball can be used to help apply pressure.

Tips for the Expectant Dad
What Can I Do? How Can I Help?

Offer to give your partner a massage or to rub her feet or back during labor. It may help her relax, or it can ease tension and soreness. However, if your partner doesn't want a massage—she might be quite vocal about it—don't push it. Always ask her *first* what she would like you to do.

Anesthesia and Analgesics

Uterine contractions and cervical dilatation during labor cause pain. As labor progresses and the baby's head moves through the birth canal, pressure on the vagina, pelvic floor and perineum also causes pain.

- There are many different types of pain relief for labor and delivery.
- *Analgesia* is pain relief without total loss of sensation.
- *Anesthesia* is pain relief with partial or total loss of sensation.
- Recent studies indicate more women are asking for pain relief during labor; one reason seems to be that effective pain relief can be achieved with smaller doses of anesthetics, which helps reduce side effects and aftereffects.
- About 66% of all women who deliver at large hospitals ask for pain relief during labor or delivery. In smaller hospitals, that number is around 42%.

Analgesia

- Analgesia is injected into a muscle or vein to decrease the pain of labor; you remain conscious.
- Examples of analgesia are Demerol (meperidine) and morphine.

- It provides pain relief but can make you drowsy, restless or nauseous.
- You may find concentration difficult.
- Analgesia may slow the baby's reflexes and breathing, so these medications are usually given during the early and middle parts of labor.

Anesthesia

- There are three types of anesthesia—general anesthesia, local anesthesia and regional anesthesia.
- You are completely unconscious under *general anesthesia,* so it is used only for some Cesarean deliveries and emergency vaginal deliveries.
- With general anesthesia, the baby is also anesthetized and needs to be resuscitated after delivery.
- An advantage of general anesthesia is that it can be administered quickly in an emergency.
- *Local anesthesia* affects a small area and is useful for an episiotomy repair.
- It rarely affects the baby and usually has few lingering effects.
- *Regional anesthesia* affects a larger body area. The three most common types of regional anesthesia are epidural block, spinal block and pudendal block.
- Epidural anesthesia is the most commonly used form of pain relief for labor and delivery in the United

States and provides the most effective pain relief during labor.

- An epidural or a spinal block, discussed below, may cause a woman's blood pressure to drop suddenly, which in turn can cause a decrease in the baby's heart rate.
- These blocks are not used if a woman is bleeding heavily or if the baby has an abnormal heartbeat.
- One other possible side effect from these two blocks is severe headache caused by leakage of spinal fluid from the puncture site.
- These headaches are treated with pain medication, lying down or drinking lots of fluid.
- Sometimes a *blood patch* is used to close the puncture site.
- With a blood patch, a small amount of your blood is withdrawn from your arm, then placed in the area of the puncture to seal the leak. It is usually very effective.

Tips for the Expectant Dad
What Can I Do? How Can I Help?

Allow and encourage your partner to use the methods she chooses for pain control. Having a baby is painful—more than any man will ever understand. If an epidural or other type of pain control is available and she chooses to use it, support her choice and help her make its use possible.

Epidural Block

- With an epidural block, a tube is inserted into a space, called the *epidural space,* outside your spinal column in the lower back.
- Medication is administered through the tube for pain relief, and you remain conscious during delivery.
- Epidural block is a procedure done during labor or for a C-section.
- It numbs the pain of contractions; it can be strong enough to allow a Cesarean delivery to be performed.
- An epidural is usually performed by an anesthesiologist (a medical doctor) or a nurse trained in the procedure (CNA or certified nurse anesthetist).
- To receive an epidural, you curve your spine and push your back out while sitting up or lying on your side.
- Antiseptic solution is used to wash your back, then the skin is numbed with a local anesthetic.
- A needle is placed in the numbed area, into your middle or lower back, near the spine in the epidural space.
- A small plastic catheter similar to an I.V. is placed in the space, and anesthetic medication is given through this catheter.
- When you need pain relief, it is given with a syringe through the catheter or the catheter is attached to a pump that gradually releases it.

- The tube remains in place until after the baby is born so medication can be readministered as necessary.
- An epidural helps relieve painful uterine contractions, pain in the vagina and rectum as the baby passes through the birth canal and the pain of an episiotomy.
- It causes some loss of, or a decrease in, sensation in the lower part of the body.
- If you have an epidural, you may feel pressure sensations with contractions so you are able to push during vaginal delivery.
- Because an epidural may make it harder to push, vacuum extraction or forceps may be necessary during delivery. See page 115 for further information.
- You may have heard that if you have epidural anesthesia during labor, you have a greater chance of having a C-section. Research shows there is *no* connection between the use of epidurals and the rate of Cesarean deliveries.
- An epidural does not lengthen the first stage of labor (from the beginning of contractions to complete dilatation at 10cm).
- If it affects your ability to push during the second stage of labor, your doctor can wait a little while and let the epidural wear off so you can push.

A *"Walking Epidural"*

- A *walking epidural,* also called *intrathecal anesthesia,* can be given to you if you suffer extreme pain in the early stages of labor (dilated less than 5cm).
- A small amount of narcotic, such as Demerol, is injected through a thin needle into the spinal fluid, which eases the pain and causes few side effects.
- Because the dose is small, neither you nor your baby becomes overly drowsy.
- Your sensory and motor functions remain intact, so you can walk around with help, sit in a chair or go to the bathroom.
- Walking epidurals may not have as much of an effect on your ability to push.
- This type of epidural is not available everywhere.

Spinal Block

- A spinal block is similar to an epidural; however, it is not usually used during labor.
- A single dose is given that lasts long enough for a Cesarean delivery to be performed or for a birth, but it doesn't last long enough for labor.

- This type of block is administered only once during labor, so it is often used just before delivery or the Cesarean section.
- A spinal is given like an epidural, but the needle is placed into the spinal canal.
- Medication is injected into spinal fluid in the lower back to numb the lower part of the body. You remain conscious.
- It provides pain relief for 1 to 2 hours.
- A spinal block works quickly and is an effective pain inhibitor.

General Anesthesia

- General anesthesia is usually used for emergency Cesarean deliveries or emergency vaginal deliveries, when there isn't time for an epidural or spinal.
- It is administered using a combination of I.V. and inhaled medications.
- If you receive general anesthesia, you are unconscious or asleep.

Other Blocks

- A *local block* provides pain relief in a localized area.
- It is given in the area between the vagina and rectum using a needle and syringe.

- It is most often used just before delivery to provide pain relief for an episiotomy and episiotomy repair.
- A *pudendal block* is medication injected into the pudendal nerve area in the vagina to relieve pain and pressure in the vaginal area, the perineum and the rectum.
- You remain conscious, and side effects are few.
- Pudendal block is considered one of the safest forms of pain relief; however, it does not relieve uterine pain or pain from contractions.

Tips for the Expectant Dad
What Can I Do? How Can I Help?

Help with the mood or environment in the labor room. This may have to do with music selection or volume, the TV or even surprise visits by family and friends. Do whatever is necessary to protect your partner's privacy and to make the experience as pleasant as possible for both of you.

When You're Overdue

Not every woman delivers by her due date. Nearly 10% of all babies are born more than 2 weeks late. A pregnancy is considered to be overdue *(postterm)* only when it exceeds 42 weeks or 294 days from the first day of the last menstrual period. (A baby that is 41 weeks and 6 days is *not* postterm!)

- Your doctor will examine you to see if your cervix is dilated and thinned, and if the baby's head is presenting.
- If the baby is healthy and active, you are usually monitored until labor begins on its own.
- Tests may be done as reassurance that an overdue baby is fine and can remain in the womb.
- These tests include a *nonstress test,* a *contraction-stress test* and a *biophysical profile.*
- They are discussed in Part I. If tests show signs of fetal stress, labor is often induced.

Keep a Positive Attitude

- It's often hard to keep a positive attitude when you're overdue, but don't give up!
- Keep eating well, and keep up your fluid intake.
- If you can do so without any problems, get some mild exercise, like walking or swimming.
- Rest and relax now because your baby will be here soon, and you'll be very busy.
- Use the time to get things ready for baby so you'll be all set when you both come home from the hospital.

- Keep your prenatal appointments, follow suggestions and don't be afraid to ask your doctor any questions you have.

Postterm Pregnancies

- Most babies born 2 weeks or more past their due date are delivered safely.
- Carrying a baby longer than 42 weeks may cause some problems for the fetus and the mother, so tests are done on these babies to make sure they are OK. Labor is induced when necessary.
- While the fetus is growing and developing inside your uterus, it depends on two important functions performed by the placenta—respiration and nutrition. The baby relies on these functions for continued support, growth and development.
- When a baby is overdue, the placenta may fail to provide the respiratory function and essential nutrients the baby needs to grow, and an infant may begin to suffer nutritional deprivation. The baby is called *postmature.*
- At birth, a postmature baby has long fingernails, abundant hair and skin that is dry, cracked, peeling and wrinkled. There also is less vernix covering the body.

- The baby appears almost malnourished, with decreased amounts of subcutaneous fat.

Tips for the Expectant Dad   *What Can I Do? How Can I Help?*

Go outside the room to eat. You partner can't eat, but she may be hungry. Imagine her having to sit and watch you or others eat during labor. Be thoughtful in all you do and say during labor and delivery.

Inducing Labor

There may come a point in your pregnancy that your doctor decides to induce labor; it's a fairly common practice. Each year, doctors induce labor for about 450,000 births. Labor is induced for overdue babies, chronic high blood pressure in the mother, pre-eclampsia, gestational diabetes, intrauterine-growth restriction and Rh-isoimmunization.

- If you are overdue, your doctor may examine you to determine if you are *favorable* for induction. See the discussion below.
- The baby is evaluated to see how it is doing. This evaluation may be done with a biophysical profile, as discussed on page 35.

- If the tests are reassuring and baby is healthy and active, you are usually monitored until labor begins on its own.

Bishop Score
(Bishop Pelvic Scoring System)

- The Bishop score is used to predict the success of inducing labor.
- The test is a method of evaluating the cervix.
- Measurements include dilatation, effacement, station, consistency and position of the cervix.
- A score of 0, 1, 2 or 3 is given for each area, then scores are added together.
- A score of 8 or more indicates the probability of a successful vaginal delivery after labor is induced and is similar to that after labor that begins on its own.
- A score of 9 or higher indicates a high chance of a successful induction of active labor.
- As the Bishop score decreases, the rate for successfully inducing labor falls.

Ripening the Cervix for Induction

- Today, doctors sometimes ripen the cervix before labor is induced.

- *Ripening the cervix* means medication is given or mechanical means are used to help the cervix soften, thin and dilate.
- Various preparations are used for this purpose.
- The two most common are Prepidil Gel (dinoprostone cervical gel, 0.5mg) and Cervidil (dinoprostone, 10mg).
- Cervidil uses a controlled-release system.
- In most cases, doctors use Prepidil Gel or Cervidil to prepare the cervix the day before induction.
- The preparation is placed in the top of the vagina, behind the cervix.
- Medication is released directly onto the cervix, which helps it to ripen (soften) for induction of labor.
- *Mechanical means* for ripening the cervix include balloon catheters and osmotic dilators (Laminaria).
- Doctors do this procedure in the labor-and-delivery area of the hospital, so the baby can be monitored.

Induction of Labor

- If your doctor induces labor, you may first have your cervix ripened, as described above, then you will usually receive oxytocin (Pitocin) intravenously.
- This medication is gradually increased until contractions begin.

- The amount of oxytocin you receive is controlled by a pump, so you can't receive too much of it.
- The oxytocin starts contractions to help you go into labor.
- While you receive oxytocin, you and your baby will be monitored for the baby's reaction to your labor.
- The length of the entire process—ripening your cervix until the birth of your baby—varies from woman to woman.
- It is important to realize that being induced or having an induction does *not* guarantee a vaginal delivery.
- In many instances, the induction doesn't work. In that case, a C-section is usually necessary.

Rupturing Membranes
(Amniotomy)

- Rupturing membranes, also called *amniotomy*, involves breaking the amniotic sac, which can stimulate contractions, if they haven't started, or make them stronger if they have already started.
- It is done in labor and delivery during a pelvic exam.
- Membranes are ruptured with an instrument called an *amni hook* (a thin plastic instrument the size of a straw) or by placing an internal fetal monitor on the baby's head.

Stripping Membranes

- Some doctors "strip membranes" to help labor start; however, this procedure is controversial and doesn't always work.
- Stripping membranes causes the release of hormones called *prostaglandins* that can cause contractions that lead to labor.
- The doctor inserts a gloved hand through the vagina and inserts a finger through the cervix. He or she then sweeps a finger between the cervix and the fetal membranes (amniotic sac).
- Stripping membranes may cause you to bleed a little and to cramp.

Can Your Baby Get Tangled in the Cord?

- Some babies can get tangled in their umbilical cord and can get the cord tied in a knot or wrapped around their neck.
- However, nothing you do during pregnancy causes or prevents this from happening.
- A tangled umbilical cord isn't necessarily a problem during labor.

- It only becomes a problem if the cord is stretched tight around the baby's neck or is in a tight knot.

Tips for the Expectant Dad   *What Can I Do? How Can I Help?*

Be part of what's going on during labor. Don't spend a lot of time on the phone, do work or otherwise try to make "good use" of your time while your partner is in labor. Be there physically and emotionally for her.

Is an Episiotomy Always Necessary?

- An *episiotomy* is an incision made from the vagina toward the rectum during a vaginal delivery.
- Many women do not want an episiotomy for the delivery of their baby because they don't think it's necessary.
- Ask your doctor at one of your prenatal visits if an episiotomy is routine or if it is done only when necessary.
- Understand that your doctor may not be able to make this decision until delivery.
- Some situations do not require an episiotomy, such as a small or premature baby.
- The more children a woman has, the less likely it is she will need an episiotomy; it also depends on the size of the baby.
- Some things that may lead to an episiotomy include the size of the mother's vaginal opening, the size of the baby's head and shoulders, the number of babies previously delivered and whether it is a forceps or vacuum delivery.

- An episiotomy is done during delivery to avoid tearing or ripping the vaginal opening or rectum, and to allow room for the baby to fit through the birth canal.

- Having an episiotomy helps avoid stretching the vagina, bladder and rectum. Stretching these areas can result in loss of control of your urine or bowels and can change sensations experienced during sexual intercourse.

- The reason for an episiotomy usually becomes clear during delivery when the baby's head is in the vagina.

- An episiotomy substitutes a controlled, straight, clean cut for a tear or rip that could go in many directions. This may include tearing or ripping into the bladder, large blood vessels or rectum.

- A surgical incision also heals better than a ragged tear.

- The area is usually washed with antiseptic soap and numbed with local anesthetic (if you don't have regional anethesia) before the incision is made.

- The cut may be made in the midline toward the rectum, or it may be a cut to the side.

- After the baby is delivered, layers are closed separately with absorbable sutures that don't need to be removed after they heal.

- Description of an episiotomy also includes a description of the depth of the incision:

  ~ a *first-degree* episiotomy cuts only the skin

~ a *second-degree* episiotomy cuts the skin and underlying tissue
~ a *third-degree* episiotomy cuts the skin, underlying tissue and rectal sphincter, which is the muscle that goes around the anus
~ a *fourth-degree* episiotomy goes through the three layers and through the rectal mucosa

- The most painful part of the entire birth experience might be an episiotomy; it may cause some discomfort as it heals.
- Don't be afraid to ask for medication to ease any pain. There are many medications that are safe to take, even if you breastfeed your baby.
- Ice, sitz baths and laxatives can also help relieve episiotomy pain.
- It gets better! Episiotomies heal and feel better within a few weeks after delivery.

Repair of an Episiotomy

- An episiotomy repair is done following the delivery of the placenta, while you are meeting your new baby.
- The episiotomy cut is repaired with sutures that are absorbed over the next few weeks.
- The two sides of the cut area are pulled together with a continuous suture.
- This procedure can take from 5 minutes to 1 hour.

Vaginal Delivery of Your Baby

Most women have a vaginal birth. There are three distinct stages of labor in a vaginal birth.

- In the first stage of labor, your uterus contracts with enough intensity, duration and frequency to cause thinning (effacement) and dilatation of the cervix. Stage one of labor ends when the cervix is fully dilated (usually 10cm) and sufficiently open to allow the baby's head to come through it.

- The second stage of labor begins when the cervix is completely dilated at 10cm and ends with the delivery of the baby. Once you are fully dilated, it's time to begin pushing. Pushing can take 1 to 2 hours (first or second baby) to a few minutes (an experienced mom). Your doctor may need to use forceps at the time of delivery, depending on the size of the baby, the size of your pelvis, how well you are able to push and whether your baby needs to be delivered immediately. Forceps are not used as much today as they were in the past. Instead, physicians more often use a vacuum extractor or perform a Cesarean section.

- The third stage of labor begins after delivery of the baby. It ends with delivery of the placenta and the membranes that have surrounded the fetus. Delivery of the baby and placenta and repair of the episiotomy usually take 20 to 30 minutes. Stitching closed the various skin and muscle layers after baby is born may take quite a bit of time.

- After your baby is born, you are both evaluated.
- You will go to recovery for a short time, then move to a hospital room until you're ready to go home.
- If your hospital has LDRP (labor, delivery, recovery and postpartum in the same room), you may stay in one room the entire time you are in the hospital.
- Your first bowel movement usually occurs a few days after delivery. It could be uncomfortable, especially if you have an episiotomy. If you had an enema, it could take a few days longer.

Tips for the Expectant Dad
What Can I Do? How Can I Help?

Be in charge of photo and video equipment. Discuss ahead of time the guidelines your partner prefers. Not every pregnant woman wants her entire delivery recorded for all to see. She may prefer not to have pictures or video taken of the more personal and private moments she experiences.

Forceps Delivery and Vacuum Extraction

- Some deliveries require assistance to help deliver the baby's head.
- Doctors use forceps and/or vacuum delivery in about 10 to 15% of all vaginal deliveries.

- This may occur if you push for a long time but the baby's head just won't deliver or if the baby is having trouble and needs to be delivered quickly.
- In some cases, *forceps* are used to help deliver the baby's head.
- Forceps look like two large salad spoons. They are inserted into the vagina and placed on either side of the baby's scalp.
- As you push, the doctor gently pulls to help deliver the baby.
- Another method is *vacuum delivery,* also called *vacuum extraction.*
- A soft plastic cup is placed on baby's head. Suction is then applied to hold the cup on baby's head.
- As you push, your doctor can gently pull on the suction cup to help deliver your baby.

A Retained Placenta

- In most instances, the placenta is delivered within 30 minutes after the birth of your baby and is a routine part of the delivery.
- In some cases, a piece of placenta or some placental membranes remain inside the uterus and do not deliver.
- When this happens, the uterus cannot contract adequately, resulting in vaginal bleeding that can be heavy.

- In other cases, the placenta does not separate because it's still attached to the wall of the uterus. This can be a very serious situation, but it is rare.
- Bleeding is often severe with a retained placenta, and surgery may be necessary to stop it.
- Reasons for an abnormally adherent placenta are many.
  - ~ It is believed a placenta may attach over a previous Cesarean-section scar or other previous incisions on the uterus.
  - ~ The placenta may attach over an area that has been scraped, such as with a D&C, or over an area of the uterus that was infected at one time.
- Some people ask to see the placenta after delivery; you may want to ask your doctor to show it to you.
- Your doctor will pay attention to the delivery of your placenta while you and your partner are paying attention to your baby.

Manual Removal of the Placenta

- Fortunately, manual removal of the placenta is not a procedure we have to do often.
- Following delivery, the placenta is usually expelled with a few contractions.
- When this doesn't happen, the placenta may have to be manually removed by your doctor.

- He or she places a hand inside the vagina far enough to reach the placenta and assists in delivering it.

D&C for a Retained Placenta

- In some cases, a D&C (dilatation & curettage) may need to be done for a retained placenta.
- This is necessary when the entire placenta doesn't deliver. Pieces of placenta or membranes can be stuck inside the uterus following delivery.
- When this occurs, bleeding can be heavy.
- A D&C is done in an operating room, either with your epidural or with general anesthesia.
- A small tube attached to a suction machine is placed into the uterus to remove the tissue.
- Removal of tissue allows the uterus to contract and to stop bleeding.

Tips for the Expectant Dad — *What Can I Do? How Can I Help?*

Continue to be supportive of your partner after baby's birth. Stay with her while the doctor stitches her episiotomy or waits for the delivery of the placenta. Together share the wonderful experience of meeting your new baby.

Cesarean Delivery

A Cesarean delivery is also called a *C-section*. When you have a Cesarean delivery, the baby is delivered through an incision made in your abdominal wall and uterus.

- There are many reasons for doing a C-section, but the main goal is to deliver a healthy baby and to preserve the health of the mother.
- The rate of C-sections done in the U.S. is between 15 and 20% of all deliveries.
- One reason for Cesarean deliveries is better monitoring during labor and safer procedures for C-sections.
- A Cesarean delivery may be necessary if your baby is too big to fit through the birth canal. This condition is called *cephalo-pelvic disproportion* (CPD).
- CPD may be suspected during pregnancy, but usually labor must begin before your doctor will know.
- A C-section may also be recommended if an ultrasound shows your baby is very large—usually at least 9 pounds, 14 ounces.
- Your doctor doesn't usually know whether you will need a Cesarean before labor begins.
- You will probably be in labor before you will know whether you will have a C-section.
- Talk to your doctor about Cesarean delivery several weeks before your due date.

- Tell your doctor your wishes and concerns in regard to having a Cesarean delivery.

How a Cesarean Is Performed

- An incision is made through the skin of the lower abdomen down to the uterus, and the wall of the uterus is cut.
- The amniotic sac containing the baby and placenta is cut, and the baby is removed through the incisions.
- After the baby is delivered, the placenta is removed.
- The uterus is closed in layers with absorbable sutures (they don't have to be removed).
- Finally, the abdomen is sewn together.
- You may have an epidural or spinal anesthetic so you stay awake. You can see and hold your baby immediately after birth, and your partner can be with you.
- A Cesarean delivery is major surgery and carries with it certain risks, including infection, bleeding, shock through blood loss, the possibility of blood clots and the possibility of injury to other organs, such as the bladder or rectum.
- Recovery is slower with a Cesarean than with a vaginal delivery. Full recovery normally takes 4 to 6 weeks.

After Your Cesarean Delivery

- You will probably stay in the hospital an extra couple of days.
- In the past, doctors usually recommended a woman have no solid food until 2 days after delivery.
- Recent research shows that this time may be cut from a few days to a *few hours* after the procedure.
- In the past, many Cesarean deliveries required general anesthesia; food is not recommended after general anesthesia.
- However, today most C-sections require regional anesthesia (epidural or spinal), so the same rules often do not apply.

Tips for the Expectant Dad

What Can I Do? How Can I Help?

If your partner has a C-section, she'll still need your support. Stay with her, even if it's just to hold her hand. You don't have to watch the surgery—nobody expects you to do more than you feel comfortable doing. You'll be glad you stayed when the doctor introduces you to your new baby.

Vaginal Birth after Cesarean (VBAC)

- One-third of all Cesarean deliveries are repeat C-sections.

- Some women who have had a C-section with one pregnancy deliver vaginally with a later pregnancy. This is called *vaginal birth after Cesarean (VBAC)*.
- A high percentage of VBAC deliveries are successful, if pregnancy and labor are closely monitored.
- There is some risk that the internal surgical scar from an earlier C-section could stretch and pull apart, called *uterine rupture,* during labor and delivery.
- This can happen if hormones are used to ripen the cervix and/or induce labor.
- One study showed that a woman's risk of uterine rupture with VBAC increased *15 times* if hormones are applied to the cervix to ripen it.
- If an intravenous hormone is used to induce labor, such as oxytocin, the risk of rupture increased *5 times.*
- Contractions may be too strong for a uterus that is scarred by previous surgery.
- Risk also increases for a woman who gets pregnant within 9 months of having a previous C-section.
- In this case, the uterus is *3 times* more likely to rupture.
- This might happen because it can take from 6 to 9 months for the uterine scar to heal (this is the scar on the uterus, not your abdomen).
- Until enough healing time has elapsed, the uterus may not be strong enough to stand up to the stress of labor contractions of a vaginal delivery.

- VBACs are safer when at least 18 months have passed between the previous C-section and the attempted vaginal delivery.
- Certain criteria must be met before you can have a VBAC, including the following.
  - ~ The type of uterine incision from the previous Cesarean delivery is important. (This incision may or may not be similar to the incision made in your abdomen.) With a classical incision, which goes high up on the uterus, labor is *not* permitted in subsequent pregnancies.
  - ~ The size of your pelvis is important. If you are small and your baby is large, it may cause problems.
  - ~ You have no medical complications, such as diabetes or high blood pressure.
  - ~ You are expecting only one baby.
  - ~ Your baby is entering the birth canal head first.
- If you are considering a vaginal birth with this pregnancy, the American College of Obstetricians and Gynecologists (ACOG) suggests the birthing facility should be able to perform an emergency C-section within 30 minutes, monitor the fetus continuously and have a fully equipped, 24-hour blood bank.
- If you are interested in VBAC, discuss it with your doctor well in advance of labor so plans can be made.

Delivering More than One Baby

- Delivering more than one baby often depends on how the babies are lying in your uterus.
- Possible complications of labor and delivery, in addition to prematurity, include the following:
  - ~ abnormal presentations (breech or transverse)
  - ~ prolapse of the umbilical cord (the umbilical cord comes out ahead of the babies)
  - ~ placental abruption
  - ~ fetal distress
  - ~ bleeding after delivery
- Because there is higher risk during labor and delivery, precautions are taken before delivery and during labor, including the need for an I.V., the presence of an anesthesiologist and the availability and possible presence of pediatricians or other medical personnel to take care of the babies.
- With twins, all possible combinations of fetal presentations can occur.
- Both babies may come head first (vertex).
- They may come breech, meaning bottom or feet first.
- They may come sideways or *oblique*, meaning at an angle that is neither breech nor vertex.
- Or they may come in any combination of the above.

- When both twins are head first, a vaginal delivery may be attempted and may be accomplished safely.
- It may be possible for one baby to deliver vaginally.
- The second one could require a C-section if it turns, the cord comes out ahead of the baby or the baby is distressed following delivery of the first fetus.
- Some doctors believe delivery of two or more babies requires a C-section.
- After delivery of two or more babies, the doctor pays close attention to maternal bleeding because of the rapid change in the size of the uterus.
- The uterus is greatly overdistended with more than one baby.
- Medication, usually oxytocin (Pitocin), is given by I.V. to contract the uterus to stop bleeding so the mother doesn't lose too much blood.
- A heavy blood loss could produce anemia and make a blood transfusion or long-term iron supplementation necessary.

Emergency Childbirth

Emergency childbirth can happen to anyone, so it's a good idea to be prepared. About 1 in 300 women delivers her baby in the car, on the way to the hospital. Read and study the information in the lists on the following pages. Be sure you have the names and telephone numbers of your doctor and those of friends or family near the phone. And if it happens to you, relax and follow the instructions provided on the following pages.

Tips for the Expectant Dad
What Can I Do? How Can I Help?

If an emergency birth happens to you and your partner, keep your cool! You must take control to help you both get through the experience. If you remain calm, it will give your partner confidence that you can handle the situation.

Emergency Delivery
If You Are Alone

1. Call 911 for help.
2. Call a neighbor, family member or friend (have phone numbers available).
3. Try not to push or to bear down.
4. Find a comfortable place, and spread out towels or blankets.
5. If the baby comes before help arrives, try to use your hands to ease the baby out while you gently push.
6. Wrap the baby in a clean blanket or clean towels; hold it close to your body to keep it warm.
7. Use a clean cloth or tissue to remove mucus from the baby's mouth.
8. Do not pull on the umbilical cord to deliver the placenta—it is not necessary.
9. If the placenta delivers on its own, save it.
10. Tie a string or shoelace around a section of the cord. You don't need to cut the cord.
11. Try to keep yourself and your baby warm until medical help arrives.

Emergency Delivery at Home

1. Call 911 for help.
2. Call a neighbor, family member or friend (have phone numbers available).
3. Encourage the woman not to push or to bear down.
4. Use blankets and towels to make the woman as comfortable as possible.
5. If there is time, wash the woman's vaginal and rectal areas with soap and water.
6. When the baby's head delivers, encourage the woman not to push or to bear down. Instead, have her pant or blow, and concentrate on not pushing.
7. Try to guide the baby's head out with gentle pressure. Do not pull on the head.
8. After the head is delivered, gently pull down on the head and pull a little to deliver the shoulders.
9. As one shoulder delivers, lift the head up, delivering the other shoulder. The rest of the baby will quickly follow.
10. Wrap the baby in a clean blanket or clean towels.
11. Use a clean cloth or tissue to remove mucus from the baby's mouth.
12. Do not pull on the umbilical cord to deliver the placenta—it is not necessary.

13. If the placenta delivers on its own, wrap it in a towel or clean newspapers, and save it.
14. Tie a string or shoelace around a section of the cord. You don't need to cut the cord.
15. Keep the placenta at the level of the baby or above the baby.
16. Keep both mother and baby warm with towels or blankets until medical help arrives.

Emergency Delivery on the Way to the Hospital

1. Stop the car; put on your flashing warning lights.
2. Try to get help, if you have a cellular phone or a CB radio.
3. Place the woman in the back seat, with a towel or blanket under her.
4. Encourage the woman not to push or to bear down.
5. When the baby's head delivers, encourage the woman not to push or to bear down. Instead, have her pant or blow, and concentrate on not pushing.
6. Try to guide the baby's head out with gentle pressure. Do not pull on the head.
7. After the head is delivered, gently pull down on the head and pull a little to deliver the shoulders.

8. As one shoulder delivers, lift the head up, delivering the other shoulder. The rest of the baby will quickly follow.

9. Wrap the baby in a clean blanket or clean towels. Clean newspapers can be used if nothing else is available.

10. Use a clean cloth or tissue to remove mucus from the baby's mouth.

11. Do not pull on the umbilical cord to deliver the placenta—it is not necessary.

12. If the placenta delivers on its own, wrap it in a towel or clean newspapers, and save it.

13. Tie a string or shoelace around a section of the cord. You don't need to cut the cord.

14. Keep the placenta at the level of the baby or above the baby.

15. Keep mother and baby warm until you can get them to the hospital or medical help arrives.

Part IV: After Your Baby's Birth

What Happens to You and Baby after the Birth?

- Things happen quickly once your baby emerges into the world.
- First, baby's mouth and throat are suctioned.
- Then the doctor clamps and cuts the umbilical cord (or your partner may cut the cord).
- If your partner wants to cut the umbilical cord after the baby is delivered, discuss it with your doctor *before* you go into labor.
- The baby is wrapped in clean blankets and may be placed on your abdomen.
- Apgar scores are recorded at 1 minute and 5 minutes after birth. See the discussion below.
- An identification band is placed on baby's wrist or ankle.
- Usually a brief physical exam or an assessment is done right after delivery.
- The baby receives drops in its eyes to prevent infection and is given a vitamin-K shot to prevent bleeding.
- You will be asked if you want your baby to receive the hepatitis vaccine. Discuss this with your doctor

before the birth; the vaccine protects your baby against hepatitis in the future.

- Once the initial evaluation is complete, the baby is returned to you so you can get to know each other.
- Later, the baby is placed in a heated bassinet for a period of time.

Tips for the Expectant Dad
What Can I Do? How Can I Help?

Offer to make some phone calls to family or friends to let them know of baby's arrival. Be sure to let your partner make the calls she wants to; ask before you start calling.

Your Baby's Apgar Score

- After your baby is born, he or she will be examined and evaluated at 1 minute and 5 minutes after delivery.
- The system of evaluation is called the *Apgar score,* which is a way to assess an infant's condition at birth.
- In general, the higher the score, the better the infant's condition at the time of birth.
- The baby is scored in five areas. Each area is scored 0, 1 or 2; 2 points is the highest score for each category.
- The top total score is 10.
- Areas scored include baby's heart rate, respiration, muscle tone, reflexes and color.

- If the heart rate is absent, a score of 0 is given. If it is slow, less than 100 beats per minute (bpm), a score of 1 is given. If it's over 100 bpm, 2 points are scored.
- Respiratory effort indicates the newborn's attempts at breathing. If the baby isn't breathing, the score is 0. If breathing is slow and irregular, the score is 1. If the baby is crying and breathing well, the score is 2.
- Muscle tone evaluates how well the baby moves. If arms and legs are limp and flaccid, the score is 0. If some movement is observed and the arms and legs bend a little, the score is 1. If the baby is active and moving, the score is 2.
- Reflex irritability is scored 0 if the baby doesn't respond to stimulus, such as rubbing his or her back or arms. If there is a small movement or a grimace when the baby is stimulated, the score is 1. A baby who responds vigorously is scored with 2 points.
- The baby's color is rated 0 if the baby is blue or pale. A score of 1 is given if the baby's body is pink, and arms and legs are blue. A completely pink baby is scored at 2.
- A perfect score of 10 is unusual. Most babies receive scores of 7, 8 or 9 in a normal, healthy delivery.
- A baby with a low 1-minute Apgar score may need to be resuscitated. This means a pediatrician or nurse must help stimulate the baby to breathe and to recover from the delivery.

- In most cases, the 5-minute Apgar score is higher than the 1-minute score because the baby becomes more active and more accustomed to being outside the uterus.

Tips for the Expectant Dad   *What Can I Do? How Can I Help?*

If your baby goes to the nursery, return often to let your partner know what is happening with the baby and how he or she is doing.

Saving Umbilical-Cord Blood

Some families choose to store their baby's umbilical-cord blood. *Cord blood* is blood left in the umbilical cord and placenta after a baby is born.

- In the past, the placenta and the umbilical cord were usually discarded following delivery.
- Today, there is a great deal of interest about saving cord blood after delivery.
- Researchers have found that stem cells, present in cord blood, have proved very useful in treating some diseases now treated with bone-marrow transplants.
- Cord blood contains the same valuable cells found in bone marrow that are the building blocks of the blood and immune systems.

- These special cells are undeveloped in cord blood, so cord blood does not need to be matched as closely for transplant as bone-marrow blood does. This can be very important for those in ethnic minority groups or people with rare blood types, who often have more difficulty finding acceptable donor "matches."
- Cord blood has been used successfully to treat childhood leukemia, some immune diseases and other blood diseases.
- Research is being done in the United States and Europe to use cord blood for gene therapy in a number of diseases, including sickle cell anemia, diabetes and AIDS.
- Before your baby's birth, you may ask about having your baby's cord blood collected and "banked" for future use.
- The blood can be used by the child from whom it was collected, his or her siblings or parents or other family members.
- You also may donate your baby's cord blood at no cost to you, similar to blood banking.
- Blood is collected directly from the umbilical cord immediately after delivery. There is no risk or pain to the mother or baby.
- Blood is then transported to a banking facility where it is frozen and cryogenically stored.

- Ask your doctor about this at a prenatal appointment—especially if your family has a history of certain diseases.
- Ask about how and where blood is stored and the cost of storing it.
- The cost of cord-blood banking can vary and includes an initial fee and a yearly storage fee.
- At this time, blood storage is not normally covered by insurance.
- However, some health-insurance companies pay the fees for families at high risk of cancer or genetically based diseases.
- Cord-blood banking services may waive fees for at-risk families who can't afford them.
- If you don't want to waste your baby's cord blood, think about donating it.
- A nonprofit bank can match it with someone who needs it.

Tips for the Expectant Dad
What Can I Do? How Can I Help?

Be in charge of crowd control in the room. Labor and delivery are exhausting and can be traumatic; neither you nor your partner will probably want a party going on. Be considerate of how your partner is doing. You may also want to spend some quiet time together getting to know your new son or daughter.

Changes You May Experience after Your Baby Is Born

You will probably be discharged from the hospital a day or two after your baby is born, if labor and delivery were normal and the baby is doing well.

- Some women choose to go home 24 hours after the birth of their baby or even sooner.
- If you have a Cesarean delivery, you need to stay a few days longer.
- Your blood pressure and bleeding are checked regularly in the first hours after the birth.
- You will be offered medication for pain relief and encouraged to nurse your baby.

Changes in the Uterus

- Your uterus goes through great changes after your baby is born; it takes several weeks for it to return to its original size.
- The size of your uterus at birth is quite large to accommodate the baby.
- After you deliver your baby, the uterus shrinks from the size of a watermelon to the size of a volleyball.
- Immediately after delivery, you can feel the uterus at the level of your navel; it should feel very hard.

- You are checked frequently to make sure your uterus remains hard after delivery. If it feels soft, you or a nurse can massage it so it becomes firm.
- The uterus shrinks about a finger's width each day; this is called *involution.*
- In the hospital, someone will check you every day; the exam can be a little uncomfortable.
- You will probably feel afterpains for several days following the birth as your uterus contracts to prevent heavy bleeding and to return to its normal size.
- Cramps may be eased by lying on your stomach and taking mild pain relievers.
- An empty bladder enables the uterus to work more efficiently, with less pain, so drink lots of fluids and urinate often.
- If you breastfeed, you may find that afterpains intensify during feedings.
- When your baby sucks, the pituitary gland is stimulated to release oxytocin, which makes the uterus contract.
- These extra contractions are good for you because they help control bleeding, but they may be uncomfortable.
- Mild pain medication can offer relief.

Bleeding after Delivery

- It is not unusual to lose blood during labor and delivery; however, heavy bleeding after the baby is born can be serious.
- A loss of more than 17 ounces (500ml) in the first 24 hours after your baby's birth, called *postpartum hemorrhage,* is significant.
- Bleeding is controlled by massaging the uterus (called *Credé*) and with medications.
- Bleeding lessens gradually over time, then stops.
- Breastfeeding helps your uterus contract, which can control bleeding even more.
- The most common causes of heavy bleeding include:
  - ~ a uterus that won't contract
  - ~ tearing of the vagina or cervix during birth
  - ~ a large or bleeding episiotomy
  - ~ a tear, rupture or hole in the uterus
  - ~ failure of blood vessels inside the uterus to compress
  - ~ retained placental tissue
  - ~ clotting or coagulation problems
- Problems with blood clotting can cause hemorrhaging. This may be related to pregnancy, or it may be a medical problem related to pregnancy.

- Bleeding following delivery requires constant attention from your doctor and the nurses caring for you.
- If bleeding becomes heavy after a few weeks, contact your doctor.
- If the amount of bleeding is not normal, medication may be prescribed.

Contraction of the Uterus after Delivery

- As your uterus shrinks immediately after delivery, the placenta detaches from the uterine wall.
- When the placenta detaches, there may be a gush of blood from inside the uterus signaling delivery of the placenta.
- After the placenta is delivered, you may be given oxytocin (Pitocin) to help the uterus contract and clamp down so it won't bleed.
- Massaging the uterus and using medications can help the uterus contract.
- The main reason a woman experiences heavy bleeding after delivering a baby is her uterus does not contract; this is called an *atonic* uterus.
- Your doctor, midwife or the nurse attending you may massage your uterus after delivery.

- They may show you how to do it so your uterus will stay firm and contracted.
- This is important so you won't lose more blood and become anemic.

Pain in the Perineum

- You may feel pain in the perineum, the area between the vagina and anus.
- The area may have been stretched, cut or torn during delivery.
- Most of the soreness should be gone in 3 to 6 weeks.
- Ice packs offer some pain relief in the first 24 hours after delivery. Ice numbs the area and helps reduce swelling.
- After 24 hours, a warm bath or a soak in a sitz tub can offer relief. Do this several times a day.
- Other remedies for perineal pain include numbing sprays, walking (to stimulate circulation), witch-hazel compresses and Kegel exercises.
- Urination may be painful; acidic urine can sting the cut area.
- You may want to urinate standing up in the shower with running water washing over the area.

- Pressure that was exerted on your urethra during delivery may also make it a bit more difficult to urinate after baby's birth. This will slowly clear up.

Bowel Movements

- It's not unusual to have sluggish bowels for a few days after your baby's birth.
- Your digestive system slows down during labor, and pregnancy and delivery can stress abdominal muscles.
- You may have had an enema or your bowel may have been emptied during the pushing phase of labor.
- Pain medication can also cause constipation.
- These factors all contribute to bowel habits that are different than normal.
- Don't worry about having a bowel movement for the first 4 or 5 days after the birth. Not having a bowel movement at this time is acceptable.
- To help your system work more efficiently, eat a diet high in fiber, and drink lots of fluid.
- Ask your doctor about laxatives and stool softeners.
- Prunes are a natural laxative—drink prune juice and eat prunes.
- If you don't have a bowel movement within a week after delivery or you become uncomfortable, call your doctor.

- An episiotomy or hemorrhoids can make a bowel movement more difficult or make you more apprehensive about having one.
- Your first bowel movement may feel as if it will rip or tear your episiotomy apart, but it won't.
- If you still have hemorrhoids after delivery, be assured they eventually shrink on their own.
- If you have problems with them, a compress of witch hazel or commercial compresses can offer relief. Ice packs may also help them shrink.

Your Breasts

- After delivery, your breasts may be sore, whether you breastfeed or bottlefeed.
- If you bottlefeed, your milk still comes in; doctors don't give medication to stop it as they did in the past.
- Your breasts fill with milk, called *engorgement.*
- Engorgement lasts a few days and can be very uncomfortable.
- You can ease discomfort by wearing a support bra or binding your breasts with a towel or an Ace bandage.
- Ice packs also help milk dry up.
- Don't empty your breasts unless you really have to because of pain—your body will replace the milk with more milk!

- Avoid nipple stimulation and running warm water over the breasts—both stimulate breasts to produce milk.
- You may find you have a mild fever with engorgement; however, this doesn't mean you have an infection.
- Acetaminophen can help reduce the fever and discomfort.

Vaginal Discharge

- After delivering your baby, you will experience a vaginal discharge similar to a heavy menstrual flow.
- This discharge, called *lochia,* lasts from 2 to 4 weeks.
- The discharge is red for the first 3 or 4 days, then turns pink, then brown and finally white or colorless at around 10 days.
- You will also have lochia if you have a C-section, although it may be less than appears with a vaginal birth.
- If the discharge is foul-smelling, remains heavy or is extremely light the first few days, tell your doctor. He or she may want to examine you.
- Research indicates that the incidence of toxic shock syndrome (TSS) occurs more often in the postpartum period.

- Because tampons are associated with TSS, don't use them to deal with lochia. Use sanitary napkins.
- If you do not breastfeed, your first menstrual period usually occurs within 6 to 8 weeks after giving birth.
- If you breastfeed, you may not have a regular menstrual period until you wean your baby.

Postpartum Warning Signs

- If you take care of yourself after delivery, you should not feel ill.
- Occasionally problems do occur.
- Refer to the list of symptoms and warning signs below.
- Call your doctor immediately if you experience:
  - ~ unusually heavy or sudden increase in vaginal bleeding (more than your normal menstrual flow or soaking more than two sanitary pads in 30 minutes)
  - ~ vaginal discharge with strong, unpleasant odor
  - ~ a temperature of 101F or more, except in the first 24 hours after birth
  - ~ chills
  - ~ breasts that are painful or red
  - ~ loss of appetite for an extended period

~ pain, tenderness, redness or swelling in the legs

~ pain in the lower abdomen or in the back

~ painful urination or feeling an intense need to urinate

~ severe pain in the vagina or perineum

Your Emotions

- Temporary emotional changes are not uncommon during the postpartum period.
- You may have mood swings, mild distress or bouts of crying. (See the discussion of postpartum distress that begins on page 154.)
- Mood changes are often a result of birth-associated hormonal changes in your body.
- Lack of sleep may also play a part in how you feel.
- Many women are surprised by how tired they are emotionally and physically in the first few months after the birth of the baby.
- Be sure to take time for yourself, and allow yourself a period of adjustment.
- Sleep and rest are essential after your baby is born.
- To get the rest you need, go to bed early when possible.
- Take a nap or rest when your baby sleeps.
- Ask for help from your partner, family and friends.

Are You Thinking about
Tying Your Tubes?

Some women choose to have their tubes tied (tubal ligation) while they are in the hospital after having their baby. The surgery involves blocking a woman's Fallopian tubes to prevent further pregnancies.

- This is an important decision, so take some time to think about it if you are interested.
- Being sterilized following delivery of a baby has some advantages.
- You're in the hospital and won't need another hospitalization.
- If you have an epidural, it's possible to use the epidural as anesthesia for a tubal ligation.
- If you didn't have an epidural, it may be necessary to put you to sleep.
- The procedure may also be done the morning after you've had your baby.
- Having a tubal ligation does not usually lengthen the time you're in the hospital.
- There are also disadvantages to having a sterilization at this time.
- Consider the procedure permanent and not reversible.
- Tubal ligations can be reversed, but it's expensive and requires a hospital stay of 3 to 4 days. Reversals

are about 50% effective, but pregnancy cannot be guaranteed.

- If you have your tubes tied within a few hours or a day after having your baby, then change your mind, you may regret having the tubal ligation.
- There are several ways to perform tubal ligation.
- Most common is a small incision underneath your bellybutton. The Fallopian tubes can be seen through this incision.
- A piece of the tube can be removed, or a ring or clip may be placed on the tube to block it.
- This type of surgery usually requires 30 to 45 minutes to perform.

Recovery from a Vaginal Birth

One of the first things you may notice while you rest in the hospital is how tired you feel.

- Take time to rest and recover while you're in the hospital, and take advantage of the "built-in" room service and babysitting provided there.
- For the first hour after delivery, the nurses will check you frequently for bleeding, pain, fever, blood-pressure problems and other warning signs while you and your partner bond with your baby.

- During this time, you will probably only be allowed ice chips and sips of water, even though you may be anxious to eat some food or to drink some fluids.
- Restricting food and drink is for your safety; if there are problems, such as heavy bleeding (postpartum hemorrhage), it is sometimes necessary to perform minor surgery, such as a D&C. It is safer for you to have an empty stomach if this procedure is necessary.
- If you had an epidural, it takes a few hours for it to wear off before you are able to get out of bed and walk around or go to the bathroom.
- Most doctors don't want you just to sit in bed; get out of bed and go for a walk when you feel up to it.
- If you had an episiotomy, your nurse will show you how to take care of the area while you are in the hospital and when you go home.
- Medication is available to help you with contractions and pain. It is not given routinely; it is ordered for you. All you have to do is ask for it.
- If you are Rh-negative, you may be given Rho-GAM.
- Passing urine may be uncomfortable, or it may hurt. Just take it easy, and take your time when you have to go to the bathroom.
- Laxatives or stool softeners may be given to you while you're in the hospital so you don't become constipated.

- Your baby's pediatrician will come to the hospital, do a physical on the baby, then see you to discuss making an appointment.
- If you have a boy, the pediatrician will talk to you about circumcision. Your signature is required if you choose to have this done.
- Friends and family will probably want to visit you in the hospital; don't be afraid to limit the time spent with visitors—either in person or on the telephone.
- Put a hold on your phone calls or hang a "Do not disturb" sign on your door when you want to rest.
- Before you leave the hospital, your doctor and pediatrician will talk to you about when you or your baby need to see them for your checkups.
- The nurses and your doctor will go over any precautions before you go home. This includes instructions about normal bleeding and what to do about pain.
- It is normal to have cramps or pain in the area of the episiotomy. This should lessen every day.
- Usually you will be given a prescription for mild pain medications; take them only if you need them.
- You may want to continue to take prenatal vitamins or iron.
- When you go home, gradually increase your activities.
- You may feel like you need to rest frequently—that's normal.

- Many women ask about driving and going up and down stairs.
- If you're still taking pain medicines or are having problems, such as dizziness, don't drive.
- It's OK to use stairs, if you don't overdo it.
- Following a normal pregnancy and delivery, most doctors suggest you come to see them 6 weeks after delivery for a postpartum checkup.
- Most doctors recommend you wait until your 6-week postpartum checkup before you begin any strenuous activity or exercise or become sexually active again.
- After 6 weeks, it's usually OK to resume routine activities, such as exercise, sexual intercourse and returning to work.

Recovering from a Cesarean Section

Recovery from a Cesarean delivery is different than recovery from a vaginal birth. You have undergone major abdominal surgery, so be prepared to take it easy for a while. While you have experienced many of the same situations as someone who has had a vaginal birth, you face some additional restrictions.

- You will be encouraged to get out of bed as soon as possible after your baby is born.
- Moving helps prevent blood clots, lung collapse and pneumonia.
- Walking helps restore body functions, such as relieving constipation and abdominal gas.
- Be careful not to strain stomach muscles; avoid lifting anything heavier than your baby.
- Although you did not deliver vaginally, you will probably experience painful uterine contractions for several days after baby's birth.
- This is normal and a sign your uterus is returning to its prepregnancy size.
- If you breastfeed, you may notice the pains when your baby nurses.
- If you are Rh-negative, you may be given Rho-GAM.
- Your baby's pediatrician will come to the hospital, do a physical on the baby, then see you to discuss making an appointment.
- If you have a boy, the pediatrician will talk to you about circumcision. Your signature is required if you choose to have this done.
- Friends and family will probably want to visit you in the hospital; don't be afraid to limit the time spent with visitors—either in person or on the telephone.
- Put a hold on your phone calls or hang a "Do not disturb" sign on your door when you want to rest.

- Before you leave the hospital, your doctor and pediatrician will talk to you about when you or your baby need to see them for your checkups.

- The nurses and your doctor will go over any precautions before you go home. This includes instructions about normal bleeding and what to do about pain.

- You will have lochia with a Cesarean delivery (see page 144), but your discharge may be lighter than lochia that follows a vaginal birth.

- Usually you will be given a prescription for mild pain medications; take them only if you need them.

- You may want to continue to take prenatal vitamins or iron.

- When you go home, gradually increase your activities.

- You may feel like you need to rest frequently—that's normal.

- Many women ask about driving and going up and down stairs.

- If you're still taking pain medicines or are having problems, such as dizziness, don't drive.

- It's OK to use stairs, if you don't overdo it.

- Once home, keep your incision clean and dry, and watch for infection.

- Infection of a Cesarean incision usually occurs 4 to 6 days after surgery.

- If any of the following signs appear, contact your doctor immediately. Signs of infection include:
  ~ redness that spreads from the edges of the incision
  ~ fever
  ~ hardness around the incision
  ~ discharge from the incision site
- Most doctors recommend you wait to get the go-ahead at your 6-week postpartum checkup before you begin any strenuous activity or exercise or become sexually active again.
- You can probably resume full activity after your 6-week postpartum checkup, if all is well.

Postpartum
Distress Syndrome

- After your baby is born, you may feel very emotional. You may even wonder if having a baby was a good idea.
- This is called *postpartum distress syndrome (PPDS)*.
- Most women experience some degree of postpartum distress.
- Many experts consider some degree of postpartum distress to be normal.
- Up to 80% of all women have "baby blues." See the discussion below.

- Baby blues usually appear between 2 days and 2 weeks after the baby is born.
- The situation is temporary and usually leaves as quickly as it comes.
- Symptoms of postpartum depression may not appear until several months *after* delivery.
- They may occur when the woman starts getting her period again and experiences hormonal changes.
- Postpartum distress syndrome can resolve on its own, but it can often take as long as a year.
- With more severe problems, treatment may relieve symptoms in a matter of weeks, and improvement should be significant within 6 to 8 months.
- Often medication is necessary for complete recovery.

Different Degrees of Depression

- The mildest form of postpartum distress is *baby blues*.
- This situation lasts only a couple of weeks, and symptoms do not worsen. See ways to handle baby blues, below.
- A more serious version of postpartum distress is called *postpartum depression (PPD)*.
- It affects about 10% of all new mothers.
- The difference between baby blues and postpartum depression lies in the frequency, intensity and duration of the symptoms.

- PPD can occur from 2 weeks to 1 year after the birth.
- A mother may have feelings of anger, confusion, panic and hopelessness.
- She may experience changes in her eating and sleeping patterns.
- She may fear she will hurt her baby or feel as if she is going crazy.
- Anxiety is one of the major symptoms of PPD.
- The most serious form of postpartum distress is *postpartum psychosis (PPP)*.
- The woman may have hallucinations, think about suicide or try to harm the baby.
- Many women who develop postpartum psychosis also exhibit signs of bipolar mood disorder, which is unrelated to childbirth.
- Discuss this situation with your physician if you are concerned.
- After you give birth, if you believe you are suffering from some form of postpartum distress syndrome, contact your doctor.
- Every postpartum reaction, whether mild or severe, is usually temporary and treatable.
- In addition, if after 2 weeks of motherhood you are just as exhausted as you were shortly after you delivered, you may be at risk of developing postpartum depression.

- It's normal to feel extremely tired, especially after the hard work of labor and delivery and adjusting to the demands of being a new mom.
- However, if your exhaustion doesn't get better within 2 weeks, contact your physician.

Causes of Postpartum Distress Syndrome (PPDS)

- A new mother must make many adjustments, and many demands are placed on her. Either or both of these situations may cause distress.
- Researchers aren't sure what causes postpartum distress; not all women experience it.
- A woman's individual sensitivity to hormonal changes may be part of the cause; the drop in estrogen and progesterone after delivery may contribute to postpartum distress syndrome.
- Other possible factors include a family history of depression, lack of familial support after the birth, isolation and chronic fatigue.
- You may also be at higher risk of suffering from postpartum distress syndrome (PPDS) if:
  - ~ your mother or sister suffered from the problem—it seems to run in families
  - ~ you suffered from PPDS with a previous pregnancy—chances are you'll have the problem again

~ you had fertility treatments to achieve this pregnancy—hormone fluctuations may be more severe, which may cause PPDS

~ you suffered extreme PMS before the pregnancy—hormonal imbalances may be greater after the birth

~ you have a personal history of depression

~ you have experienced any major life changes recently—you may experience a hormonal drop as a result

Handling the Baby Blues

- One of the most important ways you can help yourself handle baby blues is to have a good support system near at hand.
- Ask family members and friends to help.
- Ask your mother or mother-in-law to stay for a while.
- Ask your husband to take some work leave, or hire someone to come in and help each day.
- Rest when your baby sleeps.
- Find other mothers who are in the same situation; it helps to share your feelings and experiences.
- Don't try to be perfect.
- Pamper yourself.

- Do some form of moderate exercise every day, even if it's just going for a walk.
- Eat nutritiously, and drink plenty of fluids.
- Go out every day.
- Talk to your doctor about using antidepressants temporarily if the above steps don't work for you.

Dealing with More Serious Forms of PPDS

- Beyond the relatively minor symptoms of baby blues, postpartum distress syndrome can appear in two ways.
- Some women experience acute depression that can last for weeks or months; they cannot sleep or eat, they feel worthless and isolated, they are sad and they cry a great deal.
- Other women are extremely anxious, restless and agitated. Their heart rate increases.
- Some unfortunate women experience both sets of symptoms at the same time.
- If you experience any symptoms, call your doctor immediately.
- He or she may want to see you in the office, and prescribe a course of treatment.
- Do it for you and your family.

Your Postpartum Checkup

Your postpartum checkup is the last part of your complete prenatal-care program. This appointment is as important as any during your pregnancy.

- A postpartum checkup is scheduled between 2 and 6 weeks after delivery, depending on the circumstances of the birth.
- This is a good time to discuss your pregnancy, labor and delivery, and to ask questions. Ask if there are things you should know or do for successful future pregnancies.
- At your visit, your doctor will want to hear how you feel.
- If you have had headaches or experienced increased irritability or fatigue, he or she may prescribe an iron supplement.
- You will have a physical exam, similar to the one at your first prenatal exam.
- Your doctor may also do a pelvic exam.
- If you had any birth tears or incisions, he or she will examine them to see how they are healing.
- An internal exam is also done to determine if your uterus is returning to its prepregnant size and position.
- This is a good time to discuss birth control, if you haven't already made plans.

Authors' Note to Readers

We are always happy to hear from the readers of our books. You are welcome to address letters to us via our publisher, DaCapo Press, or you may send them to us by email. If you use email, we will probably be able to reply more quickly. Our email address is **yourpregnancy@juno.com**.

When you send us an email, please do not ask us medical questions about your particular situation. We are unable to reply to these letters, except to suggest you discuss your question with your own physician. We are happy to answer general questions about areas we address in our books. We are also happy to clear up any confusion regarding information we present. If you have comments or suggestions for areas to address in future books, we are always glad to receive these suggestions.

If you send us an email, please do not include any attachments. We will not open these because of the problem with viruses. In addition, we ask that you do not add us to any lists for stories, chain letters, prayers, political or other causes, charitable donations or any other lists you can think of.

We will attempt to answer your emails as quickly as possible, but please understand that with all the books we have published, we are kept busy updating them and doing research for new books. In addition, Dr. Curtis sees patients nearly every day. We'll get back to you as soon as we can!

Index

Also by Glade B. Curtis, M.D., M.P.H., OB-GYN, and Judith Schuler, M.S.

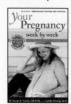

*Your Pregnancy
Week by Week, 5th Edition*
ISBN: 1-55561-346-2 (paper)
1-55561-347-0 (cloth)

*Your Pregnancy:
Every Woman's Guide*
ISBN: 0-7382-1001-3

*Bouncing Back
After Your Pregnancy*
ISBN: 0-7382-0606-7

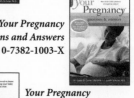

*Your Pregnancy
Questions and Answers*
ISBN: 0-7382-1003-X

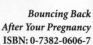

*Your Baby's First Year,
Week by Week*
ISBN: 0-7382-0975-9 (paper)
0-7382-0974-0 (cloth)

*Your Pregnancy
Quick Guide:
Feeding Your Baby in
the First Year*
ISBN: 0-7382-0968-6

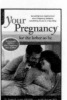

*Your Pregnancy
for the Father to Be*
ISBN: 0-7382-1002-1

*Your Pregnancy
Quick Guide:
Tests and Procedures*
ISBN: 0-7382-0953-8

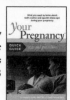

*Your Pregnancy Journal
Week by Week*
ISBN: 1-55561-343-8

*Your Pregnancy Quick Guide:
Nutrition and
Weight Management*
ISBN: 0-7382-0954-6

Your Pregnancy After 35
ISBN: 0-7382-1004-8

*Your Pregnancy
Quick Guide:
Fitness and Exercise*
ISBN: 0-7382-0952-X

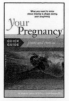

Da Capo Lifelong Books are available wherever books are sold and at special discounts for bulk purchases in the U.S. by corporations, institutions, and other organizations. For more information, please contact the Special Markets Department at the Perseus Books Group, 11 Cambridge Center, Cambridge, MA 02142, or call (800) 255-1514.